NURSING
Informatics and Technology
(Computer for Nurses)

NURSING
Informatics and Technology
(Computer for Nurses)

As per the Revised INC Syllabus for BSc Nursing

Deepak Sethi PhD (Nursing)
Professor
Sharda University
Greater Noida, Uttar Pradesh, India

Sukhbir Kaur PhD (Nursing)
Associate Professor
Department of Psychiatric Nursing
College of Nursing
Sri Guru Ram Das University of Health Sciences
Amritsar, Punjab, India

Foreword
Suresh Sharma

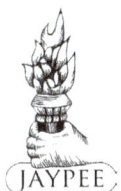

JAYPEE BROTHERS MEDICAL PUBLISHERS
The Health Sciences Publisher
New Delhi | London

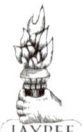 **Jaypee Brothers Medical Publishers (P) Ltd**

Headquarters
Jaypee Brothers Medical Publishers (P) Ltd
EMCA House, 23/23-B
Ansari Road, Daryaganj
New Delhi 110 002, India
Landline: +91-11-23272143, +91-11-23272703
+91-11-23282021, +91-11-23245672
Email: jaypee@jaypeebrothers.com

Corporate Office
Jaypee Brothers Medical Publishers (P) Ltd
4838/24, Ansari Road, Daryaganj
New Delhi 110 002, India
Phone: +91-11-43574357
Fax: +91-11-43574314
Email: jaypee@jaypeebrothers.com

Overseas Office
J.P. Medical Ltd
83 Victoria Street, London
SW1H 0HW (UK)
Phone: +44 20 3170 8910
Fax: +44 (0)20 3008 6180
Email: info@jpmedpub.com

Website: www.jaypeebrothers.com
Website: www.jaypeedigital.com

© 2023, Jaypee Brothers Medical Publishers

The views and opinions expressed in this book are solely those of the original contributor(s)/author(s) and do not necessarily represent those of editor(s) and publisher of the book.

All rights reserved. No part of this publication may be reproduced, stored or transmitted in any form or by any means, electronic, mechanical, photocopying, recording or otherwise, without the prior permission in writing of the publishers.

All brand names and product names used in this book are trade names, service marks, trademarks or registered trademarks of their respective owners. The publisher is not associated with any product or vendor mentioned in this book.

Medical knowledge and practice change constantly. This book is designed to provide accurate, authoritative information about the subject matter in question. However, readers are advised to check the most current information available on procedures included and check information from the manufacturer of each product to be administered, to verify the recommended dose, formula, method and duration of administration, adverse effects and contraindications. It is the responsibility of the practitioner to take all appropriate safety precautions. Neither the publisher nor the author(s)/editor(s) assume any liability for any injury and/or damage to persons or property arising from or related to use of material in this book.

This book is sold on the understanding that the publisher is not engaged in providing professional medical services. If such advice or services are required, the services of a competent medical professional should be sought.

Every effort has been made where necessary to contact holders of copyright to obtain permission to reproduce copyright material. If any have been inadvertently overlooked, the publisher will be pleased to make the necessary arrangements at the first opportunity.

Inquiries for bulk sales may be solicited at: jaypee@jaypeebrothers.com

Nursing Informatics and Technology (Computer for Nurses)

First Edition: **2023**

ISBN: 978-93-5465-824-2

Contributors

Dinesh Verma
Director
Noida International University
Greater Noida
Uttar Pradesh, India

Gagandeep Kaur
Associate Professor
Phillips School of Nursing at Mount Sinai Beth Israel
New York
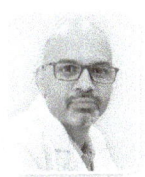

Jasneet Kaur
Associate Professor
Symbiosis International University, Pune
Maharashtra, India

Maj. Kirti Sethi
RR Hospital
New Delhi, India

Onkardeep Kaur
Lecturer
SGRD College of Nursing, SGRD University of Health Sciences, Amritsar
Punjab, India

Pawan K Sharma
Professor
Sharda University
Greater Noida
Uttar Pradesh, India

Rimple Sharma
Associate Professor
All India Institute of Medical Sciences
New Delhi, India
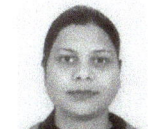

Sushma Chawla
Clinical Instructor
Rajkumari Amrit Kaur College of Nursing
New Delhi, India
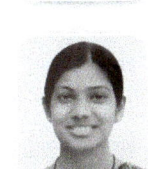

Shailza Sharma
Associate Professor
College of Nursing
Dayanand Medical College and Hospital Ludhiana,
Punjab, India
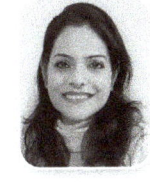

SreeRaja Kumar
Professor-cum-Vice-Principal
Sharda University Greater Noida
Uttar Pradesh, India
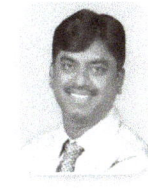

Vibha
Professor
Speciality-MCH
State Institute of Nursing and Paramedical Sciences Badal
Constituent College of Baba Farid University of Health Sciences, Faridkot
Punjab, India
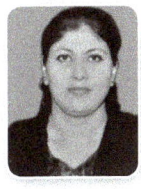

Foreword

This is an era of information and technology, where every sphere of human life is significantly influenced it. Healthcare systems and institutes including nursing sciences are significantly impacted by development of information and technology. I believe this textbook of *Nursing Informatics and Technology (Computer for Nurses)* authored by Dr Deepak Sethi and Dr Sukhbir Kaur will be reaches as a treasure on the subject and will have educative value of interpretive discussion for all students, especially in a democratic society. I also believe that teachers at every level and stage of their career can enrich and strengthen their teaching by learning the discussions, leading patterns and practices presented in this book. Participating in interpretive discussions can help teachers and students alike learn to use their minds with power and pleasure.

My experience, particularly through the COVID-19 pandemic, has been that the uniqueness of nursing informatics is the seamless integration of these three fields that leads to the effective management and communication of data, knowledge, and information within nursing practice. This textbook supports development of nursing professionals' competencies to efficiently integrate data, knowledge, and information towards fully supporting nurses, patients, payer-sources, and other key players in making decisions and playing their own roles in the continuous delivery of care. Nursing informatics is now an essential part of the Indian healthcare delivery system. In fact, the new re-envisioned Essentials of Nursing Practice state such by including two new domains of "Population Health" and "Informatics and Health Informatics Technology". As this textbook emphasizes, nursing informatics has also been lauded as a differentiating factor when it comes to selecting, implementing, and evaluating health information technology that supports top-quality and safe patient-centered care.

This edition of *Nursing Informatics and Technology (Computer for Nurses)* with its focus on improved patient outcomes using skills and knowledge for intraoperative, accurate, and meaningful healthcare data management is exactly what the industry needs. I believe the book and the associated ancillary materials support faculties who teach advanced practice registered nurses, as well as advanced practice registered nurses already in postgraduate roles. It supports these individuals by providing needed public health content and application of tools to carry out the mission. This book supports this mission because of an alignment with what is needed now. For example, when it comes to public health, it is beneficial to always share data, not just between given divisions and programs within certain departments, but also with other key agencies within the state, region, and country at large. I believe the book provides an increased skillset for professionals in nursing and the related public health informatics.

I wish both the authors a good luck!

Suresh Sharma
Professor and Principal
College of Nursing
All India Institute of Medical Sciences
Jodhpur, Rajasthan, India

Preface

Health informatics is a wide-ranging science incorporating the complex mixture of people, organizations, illnesses, patient care and treatment. It is a scientific field that deals with the storage, retrieval, sharing, and optimal use of biomedical information, data, and knowledge for problem solving and decision making. The field touches on all basic and applied fields in biomedical science and is closely tied to modern information technologies, notably in the areas 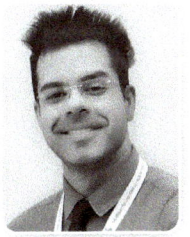 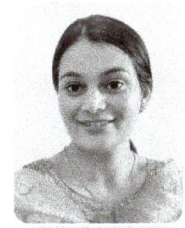 of computing and communication. Health informatics looks into ways to optimize clinical knowledge creation, sharing and application to deliver better healthcare and to promote health.

The emergence of medical informatics as a new discipline is due in large part to the rapid advances in computing and communications technologies, an increasing awareness that the knowledge base of biomedicine is essentially unmanageable by traditional paper-based methods, and a growing conviction that the process of informed decision making is as important to modern biomedicine as is the collection of facts on which clinical decisions or research plans are made.

The environments in healthcare have encompassed more than just a physical location. There is an increase in the use of technology such as mobile computers and wireless solutions, and automated exchanges between providers and patients. Adapting to these new environments requires a paradigm shift for how care is communicated and delivered, which requires knowledge of the evolution of new technologies. Nurses are at the center of this advancement as the professionals with the greatest amount of direct patient care.

We hope that this book will be of immense utility for all those for whom it is intended. We will always appreciate the comment and suggestion for improving the book.

Deepak Sethi
Sukhbir Kaur

Acknowledgment

First and foremost, we would like to thank our family members for standing beside us throughout our career and writing this book. They have been our inspiration and motivation for continuing to improve our knowledge and move our career forward. We'd like to thank our parents and grandparents for allowing us to follow our ambitions throughout our childhood. We also thank our wonderful children for always making us smile and for understanding on those weekend mornings when we were writing this book instead of playing games. We hope that one day they can read this book and understand, why we spent so much time in front of computer. We dedicate this book to all our friends and colleagues. We would like to express our gratitude to the many people who saw us through this book; to our mentors, to all those who provided support, talked things over, read, wrote, offered comments, allowed us to quote their remarks and assisted in the editing, proofreading and design. Thanks to all our friends for sharing our happiness when starting this project and following with encouragement when it seemed too difficult to be completed. We would have probably given up without their support. Sincere thanks to Dr Suresh Sharma for foreword the content of this book.

We are very grateful to the whole team of M/s Jaypee Brothers Medical Publishers (P) Ltd, New Delhi, India, who helped and guided me, Shri Jitendar P Vij (Group Chairman), Mr Ankit Vij (Managing Director), Mr MS Mani (Group President), Dr Madhu Choudhary (Director-Educational Publishing), Mr Rishi (Associate Director North, Sales and Marketing), Mr Gurdeep Singh (Executive Key Account), Ms Pooja Bhandari (Production Head), Ms Sunita Katla (Executive Assistant to Group Chairman and Publishing Manager), Ms Samina Khan (Executive Assistant to Director-Educational Publishing), Ms Alisha Talwar (Development Editor), Mr Rajesh Sharma (Production Coordinator), Ms Seema Dogra (Cover Visualizer), Mr Deep Dogra (Typesetter), Mr Rahul Jadli (Proofreader), Mr Rajesh Ghurkundi (Graphic Designer) and their team members, for all their support to work in this project and make it a success. Without their cooperation, we could not have completed this project.

Contents

1. **Introduction of Computer Application for Patient Care Delivery System and Nursing Practice** 1
   - Computer *2*
   - Application software *3*
   - Use of computer in teaching and learning *3*
   - Use of computer in research *5*
   - Use of computer in nursing practice *5*
   - Use of computer in literature search and database *6*
   - Computer databases *7*
   - Statistical packages *8*
   - Introduction to Microsoft Word *12*
   - Microsoft Excel *20*
   - Excel worksheet *20*
   - Selecting cells and ranges *21*
   - Excel features *22*
   - Microsoft PowerPoint *22*

2. **Principles of Health Informatics** 26
   - Need of nursing informatics *27*
   - Objectives of nursing informatics *27*
   - Applications of nursing informatics *27*
   - Limitations of nursing informatics *28*
   - Theories of nursing informatics *28*
   - Use of data, information and knowledge in healthcare practice *29*

3. **Information System in Healthcare** 32
   - Role and architecture of information systems *33*
   - Hospital information system *43*
   - Aims of hospital information system *45*
   - Who benefits from hospital information system? *46*
   - Subsystems of HIS *47*
   - Information system for patient care *50*
   - Clinical information system *51*
   - Systems for clinical support *52*
   - Integration of the components patient care information system *53*
   - Role of patient administration/management system *53*
   - Components of managerial information system *54*

4. **Shared Care and Electronic Health Records** 62
   - Electronic health records *63*
   - Challenges related to electronic health records implementation *65*
   - How to implement successful electronic health record system? *66*
   - Goals of electronic health records standards *67*
   - Latest trends in electronic record technology *67*

- Benefits of electronic medical records 69
- Standard for electronic health records 69

5. **Patient Safety and Clinical Risk** 73
   - Patient safety and informatics 74
   - Methods used in hospital information system for patient safety 74
   - Information technology with the greatest impact on patient safety 75
   - Future of information technology and patient safety 76
   - Risk management process 77
   - Importance of risk management in healthcare 77
   - Steps in risk management process 78
   - Applications of risk management process 81

6. **Clinical Knowledge and Decision Making** 85
   - Knowledge management system 86
   - Knowledge management methods 90
   - Health informatics standards 91

7. **E-Health: Patient and Internet** 95
   - E-health system 96
   - Use of information and communication technology to improve healthcare 97
   - Challenges in adopting e-health 99
   - Public health informatics 99

8. **Using Information in Healthcare Management** 103
   - Nursing information systems 103
   - Evaluation, analysis and presentation of healthcare data to inform decisions 113
   - Types of data analytics 114
   - Data management 115
   - Data management process 116
   - Data analysis 119
   - Data interpretation 121
   - Healthcare data in decision making 122
   - Various approaches to decision making 122
   - Challenges in healthcare data analytics 124

9. **Information Law and Governance in Clinical Practice** 128
   - Ethical legal issues in healthcare informatics 129
   - Ethics resources used in health informatics 130
   - Ethical legal issues related to digital health applied to nursing 131

10. **Healthcare Quality and Evidence-based Practice** 134
    - Evidence-based quality improvement 135
    - Role of nurse in quality improvement through EBP 137
    - Healthcare data standards 138
    - Purposes of health informatics standards 138
    - Development of healthcare standards 139

Index 143

INC Syllabus

Nursing informatics and technology

PLACEMENT: II SEMESTER

THEORY: 2 Credits (40 hours)

PRACTICAL/LAB: 1 Credit (40 hours)

DESCRIPTION: This course is designed to equip novice nursing students with knowledge and skills necessary to deliver efficient informatics-led health care services.

COMPETENCIES: On completion of the course, the students will be able to
- Develop a basic understanding of computer application in patient care and nursing practice.
- Apply the knowledge of computer and information technology in patient care and nursing education, practice, administration and research.
- Describe the principles of health informatics and its use in developing efficient healthcare.
- Demonstrate the use of information system in healthcare for patient care and utilization of nursing data.
- Demonstrate the knowledge of using Electronic Health Records (EHR) system in clinical practice.
- Apply the knowledge of interoperability standards in clinical setting.
- Apply the knowledge of information and communication technology in public health promotion.
- Utilize the functionalities of Nursing Information System (NIS) system in nursing.
- Demonstrate the skills of using data in management of health care.
- Apply the knowledge of the principles of digital ethical and legal issues in clinical practice.
- Utilize evidence-based practices in informatics and technology for providing quality patient care.
- Update and utilize evidence-based practices in nursing education, administration, and practice.

COURSE OUTLINE

T – Theory, P/L – Lab

Unit	Time (Hrs) T	Time (Hrs) P/L	Learning Outcomes	Content	Teaching/ Learning Activities	Assessment Methods
I	10	15	Describe the importance of computer and technology in patient care and nursing practice	**Introduction to computer applications for patient care delivery system and nursing practice** • Use of computers in teaching, learning, research and nursing practice	• Lecture • Discussion • Practice session • Supervised clinical practice on EHR use • Participate in data analysis using statistical package with statistician	(T) • Short answer • Objective type • Visit reports • Assessment of assignments
			Demonstrate the use of computer and technology in patient care, nursing education, practice, administration and research.	• Windows, MS office: Word, Excel Power Point • Internet • Literature search • Statistical packages • Hospital management information system	Visit to hospitals with different hospital management systems	(P) Assessment of skills using checklist
II	4	5	Describe the principles of health informatics	**Principles of Health Informatics** • Health informatics– needs, objectives and limitations • Use of data, information and knowledge for more effective healthcare and better health	Lecture Discussion Practical session Work in groups with health informatics team in a hospital to extract nursing data and prepare a report	(T) • Essay • Short answer • Objective type questions • Assessment of report
			Explain the ways data, knowledge and information can be used for effective healthcare			
III	3	5	Describe the concepts of information system in health	**Information Systems in Healthcare** • Introduction to the role and architecture of information systems in modern healthcare environments • Clinical Information System (CIS)/ Hospital information System (HIS)	• Lecture • Discussion • Demonstration • Practical session • Work in groups with nurse leaders to understand the hospital information system	(T) • Essay • Short answer • Objective type
			Demonstrate the use of health information system in hospital setting			

INC Syllabus

Unit	Time (Hrs) T	Time (Hrs) P/L	Learning Outcomes	Content	Teaching/ Learning Activities	Assessment Methods
IV	4	4	Explain the use of electronic health records in nursing practice Describe the latest trend in electronic health records standards and interoperability	**Shared Care and Electronic Health Records** • Challenges of capturing rich patient histories in a computable form • Latest global developments and standards to enable lifelong electronic health records to be integrated from disparate systems.	• Lecture • Discussion • Practice on simulated EHR system • Practical session • Visit to health informatics department of a hospital to understand the use of EHR in nursing practice • Prepare a report on current EHR standards in Indian setting	(T) • Essay • Short answer • Objective type (P) • Assessment of skills using checklist
V	3		Describe the advantages and limitations of health informatics in maintaining patient safety and risk management	**Patient Safety and Clinical Risk** Relationship between patient safety and informatics Function and application of the risk management process	Lecture Discussion	(T) • Essay • Short answer • Objective type
VI	3	6	Explain the importance of knowledge management Describe the standardized languages used in health informatics	**Clinical Knowledge and Decision Making** • Role of knowledge management in improving decision-making in both the clinical and policy contexts • Systematized Nomenclature of Medicine, Clinical Terms, SNOMED CT to ICD-10-CM Map, standardized nursing terminologies (NANDA, NOC), Omaha system.	• Lecture • Discussion • Demonstration • Practical session • Work in groups to prepare a report on standardized languages used in health informatics • Visit health informatics department to understand the standardized languages used in hospital setting	(T) • Essay • Short answer • Objective type

INC Syllabus

Unit	Time (Hrs) T	Time (Hrs) P/L	Learning Outcomes	Content	Teaching/ Learning Activities	Assessment Methods
VII	3		Explain the use of information and communication technology in patient care	**eHealth: Patients and the Internet** • Use of information and communication technology to improve or enable personal and public healthcare	• Lecture • Discussion • Demonstration	• Essay • Short answer • Objective type • Practical exam
			Explain the application of public health informatics	• Introduction to public health informatics and role of nurses		
VIII	3	5	Describe the functions of nursing information system	**Using Information in Healthcare Management** • Components of Nursing Information System (NIS) • Evaluation, analysis and presentation of healthcare data to inform decisions in the management of health-care organizations	• Lecture • Discussion • Demonstration on simulated NIS software • Visit to health informatics department of the hospital to understand use of healthcare data in decision making	(T) • Essay • Short answer • Objective type
			Explain the use of healthcare data in management of health care organization			
IX	4		Describe the ethical and legal issues in healthcare informatics	**Information Law and Governance in Clinical Practice** • Ethical-legal issues pertaining to healthcare information in contemporary clinical practice • Ethical-legal issues related to digital health applied to nursing	• Lecture • Discussion • Case discussion • Role play	(T) • Essay • Short answer • Objective type
			Explains the ethical and legal issues related to nursing informatics			

Unit	Time (Hrs) T	Time (Hrs) P/L	Learning Outcomes	Content	Teaching/ Learning Activities	Assessment Methods
X	3		Explain the relevance of evidence-based practices in providing quality healthcare	**Healthcare Quality and Evidence Based Practice** Use of scientific evidence in improving the quality of healthcare and technical and professional informatics standards	• Lecture • Discussion • Case study	(T) • Essay • Short answer • Objective type

SKILLS

- Utilize computer in improving various aspects of nursing practice.
- Use technology in patient care and professional advancement.
- Use data in professional development and efficient patient care.
- Use information system in providing quality patient care.
- Use the information system to extract nursing data.
- Develop skill in conducting literature review.

CHAPTER 1

Introduction of Computer Application for Patient Care Delivery System and Nursing Practice

At the end of this chapter, student will able to learn about:

- Characteristics of computer
- The components of computer
- Use of computer in teaching and learning
- Use of computer in research
- Use of computer in nursing practice
- Use of computer in literature search and database
- Statistical packages
- Types of statistical packages
- Statistical Package for Social Sciences (SPSS)
- Introduction to Microsoft Word
- Introduction to Microsoft Excel
- Introduction to Microsoft PowerPoint
- Hospital information system (Refer Chapter 3)

TERMINOLOGIES

- **Computer:** A computer is an electronic device that can collect data (input), process the data according to predetermined rules, produce information (output), and store the information for later use. It is controlled by instructions stored in its own memory.
- **Data:** Facts and figures that convey a specific message but are not arranged in any way and don't offer any more details about patterns, context, etc. Data, then, is defined as "unstructured facts and figures that have little to no impact on the typical manager."
- **Information:** Data must be contextualized, categorized, computed, and compacted before it can be considered information. Information, which is data with meaning and purpose, thus creates a wider picture. It could represent a trend in the market or possibly show a sales pattern over a specific time period. Essentially, answers to queries using the phrases "who, what, where, when, and how many" are where information can be obtained.
- **Knowledge:** Knowledge indicates expertise and understanding and is strongly related to doing. Each person has knowledge that stems from his or her experience and includes the standards by which they assess fresh inputs from their environment.

- **Access tool:** A device that makes it easier to find pertinent references, like a catalogue or index.
- **Statistics:** It is a vast mathematical field that researches how to gather, compile, and make inferences from data. It serves as a "collection of numerical facts or data," to put it another way.
- **Statistical package:** It is software used for gathering, organizing, interpreting, and presenting numerical data.

COMPUTER

A computer is an electronic device or equipment that receives data via a keyboard, processes it in a CPU, and outputs the desired results or information through output devices (monitor or printer).

Characteristics of a Computer

Accuracy: Despite being a machine, a computer always gives accurate results. It never makes a mistake because it generates the desired information based on the data we provide. If we properly programmed it, it will produce the most accurate response. Because of this, the phrase "GIGO" (Garbage In, Garbage Out) is used to refer to computer accuracy.

Speed: A computer executes the given instructions in billionth or trillionth of a second.

Storage: A computer is capable of holding a lot of data. A single PC may hold all of the information for an entire office, and it can rapidly retrieve any portion of the information. You can store 1.44 MB, or roughly 500 pages of text, on a floppy disc. You can store 700MB on a CD, which is 700 times more data than you can on a floppy. 500GB of data, or all the information on a large office, can be stored on a hard drive.

Multitasking: A computer is capable of doing a wide range of tasks, from document processing to satellite launch. Numerous sorts of software or applications make it feasible. A computer can perform multiple tasks sim ultaneously without slowing down. You can manage more than 40 people at once on a single computer.

Automation: Once the data and instructions are fed into a computer, normally, no human intervention is necessary during processing.

Components of a Computer

The main components of a computer are:
- Hardware
- Software

Hardware: In contrast to the intangible software components, hardware refers to the different tangible parts that make up a computer system. Although the majority of these physical parts are logically and physically segregated from the primary circuitry that does arithmetic and logical processing, these are the parts of a computer that most people are familiar with the visible and touchable parts of a computer, whether they are mechanical, electrical, or electronic, such as a keyboard or mouse.

Software: Software is a term used to describe the electronic instructions used to control a computer, carry out certain activities, and change data. Software (the instructions) needs to be programmed in order for them to carry out different tasks. In other words, the instructions

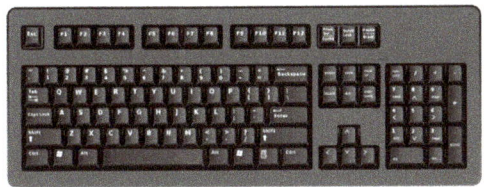
Keypad

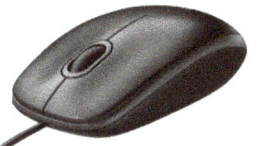
Mouse

must be written in a language that a computer can comprehend. A computer is useless without a programme. The software is a set of instructions that tells the computer how to interpret the input in addition to the physical devices.

APPLICATION SOFTWARE

Application software includes programs that users access to carry out work. They include applications for the following functions:
- The most popular software application is word processing. The main benefit of using word processing over a typewriter is that modifications may be made without having to start over from scratch. Document formatting and manipulation are made simple by word processors. For instance, WordPad, PageMaker, and MS Word.
- Spreadsheets are created and modified electronically by users of spreadsheet computer programmes (tables of values arranged in rows and columns with predefined relationships to each other). For mathematical computations, such as finances, budgets, statistics, and more, spreadsheets are used. VP Planner, for instance, or MS Excel.
- Computer programmes called database management apps allow users to create and modify data in a database. A database is a grouping of connected data that can be sorted, subjected to statistical analysis, or utilized to produce reports. Dbase, FoxPro, access, oracle, SQL server, etc. are a few examples.
- Presentation graphics and packages are computer tools that let users design highly stylized pictures for reports and slide presentations. They can also be used to create other kinds of graphs and charts. Applications for desktop publishing, paint programmes, and other graphic-based software are only a few examples. PowerPoint, as an example.

USE OF COMPUTER IN TEACHING AND LEARNING

Students can use computers to make their life easier, which is only one of the many advantages they have in education. Find out how computers are used in education.
- **Convenience:** A student's life has become quite convenient thanks to computers. Students can write and research their schoolwork online, collaborate with classmates and teachers through email or other platforms, and share knowledge with others simply by using this tablet. Indeed, a computer greatly facilitates the lives of students.
- **Improved student performance:** It is crucial that computers be used in the classroom as a tool for learning. Students are more likely to enjoy studying when they utilize computers, which leads to improved performance. When computers are being used, they feel more engaged and attentive. The use of computers in the classroom allows each student to collaborate while also teaching them to be independent.
- **Fast access to research and information:** The days of using the library as your only resource for research and assignment completion are long gone. Today, accessing all the information

you need for research is much simpler and quicker thanks to the availability of computers in schools. You may find all the information you require for your school projects in a matter of clicks.
- **Online resources:** Technology aids students in finding the most pertinent and reliable material while choosing a topic for their thesis or essay. The internet and computer technology supply all the most recent information about choosing the best thesis topic and the pertinent information to support the choice, regardless of whether the subject is science, commerce, sociology, or any other course with a name.
- **Increased efficiency:** Without a doubt, computers help every student be more productive. They can use these even beyond school hours to finish assignments, check grades, and give presentations. There are a lot of things to study, therefore the flexibility and efficiency that computers provide pupils are worth it.
- **Admissions information:** Students may easily obtain all the information they need online when they are attempting to determine which college or university to apply to. This material includes details on the admissions process as well as facts about various universities. Colleges and universities have a strong online presence. They are available to help students with practically anything they need, including questions about admissions, help with the application and visa processes, payment, and getting ready to arrive. It has benefited students and broadened the appeal of universities and other institutions, bringing in the top applicants from all over the world.
- **Study schedules:** Students need to view current information and updates while deciding which courses to take, and technology may help them do so. In this way, learners may determine the appropriate course dates; the assignment outlines also assist them in planning out their academic work.
- **Better opportunities:** Students have access to a wide range of options because to technology and the internet combined. In this way, people may learn all about them, choose what will best support their goals and success, and make an informed decision. Through messengers, they can communicate with and learn from other specialists.
- **Easy communication:** The introduction of computers has facilitated communication, particularly for students who live distant from their family. Even while they are away from home, students may easily stay in touch with their loved ones thanks to instant messaging, emails, live updates, and sharing options. Simply said, the internet and computers keep the world connected despite their distance.
- **Better rate of learning:** Thanks to technology, especially in the sciences, what used to require years of study can now be finished in a matter of seconds. There is software available now that simulates plant growth under particular conditions. The National Library of Medicine and National Institutes of Health of the US government support this kind of virtual simulation as an excellent tool for growth modeling research. Because of virtualization models, it may be said that technology helps students learn more in a shorter amount of time.
- **Visualization tools:** Many children struggle to visualize the concepts being taught, which makes arithmetic challenging for them. Students can now use applications to view relationships on the computer screen in front of them. Excuse the pun, but they get what I'm getting about. On the National Library of Virtual Manipulative, a team from Utah State University has compiled a lengthy list of arithmetic tools organized by grade/developmental stages. Students enter data, and as the data changes, the chart in front of them moves. There is no denying the fact that abstract ideas are frequently difficult to picture. With these

Introduction of Computer Application for Patient Care Delivery System and Nursing Practice

instruments, the ideas become less abstract and more concrete because they are perfectly present in front of you.
- **Making tasks easier:** Nowadays, most schools give out iPads or Chromebooks rather than expensive, bulky textbooks. They have access to all subjects, worksheets, and assignments on a small device that weighs less than two or three pounds and is portable wherever they go. Due to the fact that they upload each assignment to the cloud as it is finished, students can no longer utilize the defense that they "lost my assignment in my desk" or "I left my homework at home." To complete the assignment, all students have to do is sign into their student account, select the task, and tab to the relevant file. The sole defence is that they forgot their computer at home; if the school offers internet access, this would definitely prevent them from using social media during lunch.

USE OF COMPUTER IN RESEARCH

We frequently forget the transformative impact that computers have had on society because they are such ubiquitous components of our daily lives. Computers created new possibilities for data processing in scientific and social scientific research, generating significant knowledge and information.
- **Internet:** It's common to desire to quickly educate yourself about potential problems or study topics by examining the informational resources at your disposal before you begin your investigation. Academic journals are almost all available online, and many of them are arranged into databases. You may typically get economic or demographic data from government organizations online to help in your research.
- **Information storage:** Large volumes of data are stored in computers. Information may be organized and searched quickly and effectively, making retrieval simpler than with paper storage. Your raw data can be kept in a variety of forms. Many times using surveys, some researchers perform their study online.
- **Computational tools:** Powerful calculators were the foundation of computers, and today's research relies heavily on that function. No matter how much data you have, a computer can help you accomplish more with it. Computers have made statistical software, modeling software, and spatial mapping tools all possible. Researchers can find new patterns in how individuals use their environment by stacking various types of maps on top of one another, for example, to use information in novel ways.
- **Communication:** Research needs collaboration amongst specialists to identify new topics that need investigation and to discuss findings. This was accomplished before computers through papers and workshops. Experts from around the globe can now communicate via email or webchats. Virtual conferences can be used to convey information. Knowledge from underrepresented groups, including African scholars, is now more widely recognized.
- **Mobility:** Computers are portable, enabling researchers to collect data and perform field study more easily. The portability of computers has made it possible to conduct new types of research in isolated locations or at the local level. Websites for social media have emerged as a new way of communication and information.

USE OF COMPUTER IN NURSING PRACTICE

In order to oversee and carry out patients' healthcare plans, nurses collaborate closely with physicians and other medical specialists. Nurses in today's healthcare facilities must be well-versed in the usage of computers in the nursing field. Most of the time, medical staff no longer has to interpret written doctor's orders and patient needs from a bedside medical chart. By removing the majority of misunderstandings of verbal and written directives, electronic health records facilitate more effective communication between physicians and nurses. Nurses can develop and manage electronic health records and update them as necessary using computers, smartphones, and tablets.

- **Diagnosis:** Medical personnel can more easily collect, retrieve, and manage patient data for precise diagnosis thanks to electronic health records. Routine health examinations by nurses frequently include checking blood pressure, oxygen saturation, and even EKGs. When nurses have the technological know-how to electronically preserve the readings and store them in a patient's electronic health record, the findings of these evaluations can be recorded with more accuracy. Physicians won't need to visit the patient's room as often to retrieve diagnostic information once the records have been gathered and recorded because they will be instantly accessible to the complete patient care team. With the help of modern technology, nurses may now easily access important medical resources and nursing tools online, which speeds up and improves diagnosis.
- **Treatment and medication:** Nurses now record and examine prescription drugs in electronic health records. They handle patient meds using software and applications as well. These tools aid nurses in avoiding prescription mistakes as well as unwanted drug interactions. When a medical facility gives a patient an identifying number, nurses can access the patient's medical file and check medication orders before dispensing any prescriptions. They also provide documentation of the care given and offer advice on how to treat patients. Instead of using paper charts and whiteboards, software and electronic device apps enable nurses to update patient data using diagnostic and treatment codes. Using computer security technology also enables nurses to protect patient information.
- **Telemedicine:** Rural locations and some underserved metropolitan populations in the United States now have reduced overall access to high-quality healthcare due to ongoing nursing staff shortages. However, telemedicine gives these groups the opportunity to speak with nurses about their health concerns, who can advise them on whether or not they require treatment at a hospital. Seniors and patients with disabilities, for whom a trip to the doctor is frequently difficult, might also benefit from telemedicine. To help patients over the phone, nurses require technology that allows them to type their recommendations into a programme or enter them into the patient's medical file. To communicate with other members of the patient's care team and family, nurses can use software or an app.

USE OF COMPUTER IN LITERATURE SEARCH AND DATABASE

The amount of time that any user has for reading scientific and technical literature has largely remained constant, despite the exponential growth of this content. Clearly, no researcher knew everything, in contrast to his forebears who were experts. Worth in their area of expertise and is knowledgeable about the most recent developments advancements in his area of expertise. To be informed about such changes, he frequently requires the assistance of information experts and computer.

Steps Literature Search

The process of doing a successful literature search involves various factors. The first and most important step is to define the goal, range, depth, and precise area of the investigation.

A conversation between the user and the information specialist may be necessary. A quick evaluation of the nature and scope of the inquiry will reveal whether the search is for specific factual information, which is typically needed by a technical worker, or for a limited number of specific references, which is usually sufficient for an administrator or policy maker, or for a thorough bibliographical search, which is typically needed by a research worker. After completely comprehending a query's parameters, an appropriate search strategy should be created.

Searching through a bibliography, an encyclopedia, or a review magazine is a fantastic way to start your literature search. This offers some helpful background information as well. After completing this initial search, further research should be done using secondary sources such abstracting and indexing services.

Depending upon the topic, any one of the following situations may arise:
- There are secondary magazines on the topic.
- There are secondary journals on the topic as well as on the area surrounding it.
- There are publications on a wider range of topics but no secondary periodicals on the topic.
- There are no secondary periodicals on the topic or a related topic.

Search in Secondary Sources

When secondary periodicals on the subject and the broader subject are both available, the search must start with the secondary periodical on the specific subject and be complemented with references gathered from the periodicals covering the broader subject. The secondary periodicals that cover broader topics typically cover ancillary publications that are occasionally somewhat unrelated to the core subject of the search. But it is a well-known truth that knowledge on a specific topic can be found scattered widely across a wide range of magazines covering core, peripheral, and unrelated fields. Since, there is a significant diversity in the pattern of entry arrangement and indexing techniques, skills for consulting secondary periodicals must be developed.

COMPUTER DATABASES

As would be evident from the foregoing description should make it clear that literature search is primarily a process of information retrieval. Calvin Mooers first used the term "Information Retrieval" in 1950 and defined it as the "searching and retrieval of information from storage, according to specification by subject." In the process of communication between people, information retrieval is the goal. The following steps are included in the communication process:
- Information collection
- Selection for inclusion in the system
- Classification
- Indexing
- Dissemination
- Storage for future recovery
- Retrieval

Indexing and Abstracting Databases

A review of the development of indexing and abstracting services over time would reveal that, over the past 200 years, these services have worked to support the aforementioned information exchange process. The resources and capabilities of these information communication networks were under a great deal of stress due to the accelerating pace and perplexing complexity of information generation. However, the introduction of computers in the 1950s, their uses, and advancements in communication technology have all greatly aided in the improvement of document access and bibliographical control. These advancements have made machine-readable records particularly useful as databases, allowing users to get the necessary information much more quickly. These databases are accessible through networks, which the libraries can use to search on their own computers and those of large corporations like Lockheed (DIALOG) and System Development Corporation (ORBIT). There are now improved access chances to global literature production in a specific discipline due to the availability of such huge databases and their use for conducting literature searches through networks and vendors.

Online Searching

When online and comprehensive search is required, online searching is especially beneficial and often used. Another benefit of searching online is the ability to use BOOLEAN logic, which enables you to narrow or broaden your search as needed. By adjusting the search method, it is feasible to coordinate the pertinent terms according to the three logical operations represented by the symbols OR, AND, and NOT. In contrast to a manual search, an online search guarantees enhanced, rapid, and precise access.

The computer databases available for online searching are: (i) MEDLINE, (ii) CA Search, (iii) INSPEC, (iv) COMPENDEX, and (v) BIOSIS.

STATISTICAL PACKAGES

The ability to translate observations into numbers has evolved as one of the characteristics of the modern world. Statistics is the science that deals with numbers. In order to generate information, it crunches the statistics and arranges them intelligently. As knowledge increases as a result of this information, development continues. Computing innovations have been useful in this regard since they make it easier to complete this aspect of work accurately, quickly, effectively, and convincingly. In the statistical analysis, computers can be a huge aid. There are many different statistical tools, and it is important to determine how they are actually used. Numerous statistical processes necessitate a great deal of prior knowledge and understanding even when using a statistical software. Statistical packages are collections of software designed to aid in statistical analysis and data exploration.

Definition

It is common to refer to statistics as a "collection of numerical facts or data." The phrase "body of procedures and techniques for interpreting numerical data" is also used to refer to it. Statistical techniques serve a variety of functions, including approaches and processes for summarizing, simplification, reduction, and presentation of unprocessed data. Next, it generates predictions, tests hypotheses, and extrapolates traits of a population based on traits of a sample.

Software for gathering, organizing, interpreting, and presenting numerical data is known as a statistical package. The intricacy of calculations required to draw conclusions from the data has led to a requirement for a statistical programme. The development of computing technology has given statistics even more power.

According to **Ripley (2004),** "The most widely used piece of statistical packages/software for statistics is Excel. SPSS and SAS dominate certain communities, and Minitab is widely used in teaching.

Functions of Statistical Packages

Many people want to do research using statistical methods. Using data to support your assertions is unquestionably a good strategy. Numerous functions of statistics can be generically categorized as follows:

- **Summarize and describe data:** Data summaries and descriptions are used to enable data visualization at a glance. Cross-tabulations and graphs are created for nominal or ordinal data; z-scores are computed for interval or ratio data.
- **Variance and distribution of the data:** For nominal and ordinal data, one creates tables, charts, and graphs; for interval and ratio data, one creates box plots with interquartile ranges or histograms with normal curves.
- **Comparing groups:** When two or more populations must be compared, cross-tabulations for nominal or ordinal data and hypothesis testing for segmented continuous or numeric data are used.
- **Identify relationships:** Relationships can be found using cross-statistical packages tabulations for nominal and ordinal data, correlation coefficient calculations and scatter plots for interval and ratio data, or linear regression or ANOVA for data with one dependent variable and two or more predictor variables.
- **Determine clusters of related cases:** The issue of identifying groupings of related cases or k-means cluster analysis is resolved by performing hierarchical cluster analysis. Discriminant analysis is used to pinpoint traits of established groups.
- **Determine groups of related variables:** The goal of factor analysis is to find clusters of related variables.

Types of Statistical Packages

Software for statistical analysis, often known as statistical software, is used to collect and analyze data in order to uncover patterns and trends using scientific methods. They frequently undertake data science using statistical analysis approaches and theories, such as regression and time series analysis.

Statistical Package for Social Sciences (SPSS)

IBM's SPSS statistics is statistical software that can swiftly analyze massive data sets to produce insights for analysis and decision-making. Additionally, it can estimate and find missing values in data sets, enabling more precise reporting.

With its ability to handle massive amounts of data and many user licences, SPSS statistics is scalable and flexible and can do anything from simple statistical simulations to deep descriptive analytics. Utilizing geographic information in your analyzes will allow you to enhance your data.

Benefits
- **Data collection:** Collect all of your data because SPSS statistics can read and write to databases, spreadsheets, Microsoft Excel, and access files as well as ASCII text files. By smoothly incorporating data from different statistics packages, the tool aids in the formation of an entire picture.

- **Data preparation:** In a single step, automated data preparation may identify missing or incorrect values and clean up enormous data sets. With its data conditioning procedure, SPSS statistics enables data analysis with better precision.
- **Predictions:** The platform may be customised to your needs, leading to better predictions over time. To find potential correlations between variables, SPSS employs time-series analysis, forecasting, temporal causal modeling, and neural networks.

Statistical Software Suite (SAS/STAT)

It is a cloud-based platform for data visualization and analysis using statistical analytic methods. The programme is used by business analysts, statisticians, data scientists, researchers, and engineers to identify patterns and trends in data through statistical modeling. Its processes are multithreaded, carrying out many tasks at once, increasing analytical speed and efficiency.

Benefits
- **Accelerate decision-making:** By facilitating easy data access and taking care of data quality issues, SAS/STAT plugs gaps in the data-to-decision life cycle. The tool increases the organization-wide adoption of Hadoop by simplifying it for all users.
- **Analyze smarter**: SAS/STAT performs intelligent data analysis based on the kind and volume of the data. It analyzes big datasets with high-performance statistical modeling, evaluates tiny data sets with precise procedures, and aids in the completion of missing values with contemporary analysis approaches.
- **Access support:** To assist you in starting with the solution, SAS provides how-to videos and online documentation with examples in addition to a free e-learning course. By contacting technical assistance online groups, you can find solutions to problems and answers to questions.

Stata

Data manipulation, exploration, visualization, and statistical analysis are all possible with Stata, a statistical tool made specifically for data scientists. Stata has a graphical user interface and command-line architecture, making it usable by anyone with or without programming experience.

Behavioral science, education, medical research, economics, political science, public policy, sociology, finance, business, and marketing are just a few of the disciplines where researchers use the programme. The text, marks, margins, and other graphic components can all have different sizes.

Benefits
- **Fit-to-size version:** Choose a fit-to-size version from the four options available, depending on the size of the data set being examined and the amount of RAM.
- **Future prepration:** Stata can help you foresee the future and make preparations for it. With the use of its lasso tools, you may classify groups and patterns, forecast outcomes, and apply inferential statistics to data.
- **Work with any version:** Stata's inherent versioning functionality enables older scripts and applications to continue to function in platform updates.

- **Data import/export:** You can import and export data from a variety of sources, including text, ASCII files, spreadsheets, XLS, CSV, and SQL sources. Stata is compatible with other well-known statistical programmes since it can import files from SAS or SPSS.

Minitab

A statistics tool called Minitab offers data analytics, visualizations, and statistical analysis to help in data-driven decision making. From small to huge datasets, it can analyze them all, and by automating statistical calculations and graph construction, it enables targeted data analysis. Menus, toolbars, preferences, profiles, and sophisticated programming macro capabilities can all be customized in Minitab. Currently, only Windows or Mac operating systems can use the solution.

Benefits

- **Prepare data:** Minitab eliminates the tedious labour of data preparation by allowing you to sort through and transpose your data using a simple, one-click import process.
- **Gain more understanding:** Minitab uses cutting-edge machine learning and predictive analytics techniques to delve deeper into the data. You can get a sneak preview of what's to come by using tools for logistic regression, time series analysis, factor analysis, and cluster variables.
- **Technical support and documentation:** Technical support and documentation are provided by Minitab, who also provides a free Quick Start guide that walks you through the platform's key features and navigation. Additionally, the supplier offers animated lessons and practical exercises that are offered as distinct Quality Trainer e-Learning courses. On the Minitab website, there is also a wealth of technical material, manuals, blogs, and webinars.

GraphPad Prism

A statistics and data analysis tool specifically designed for scientific research is GraphPad prism. In the life sciences, biotechnology, healthcare and pharmaceuticals, automotive, technology, and telecom industries, researchers employ the software's statistical functions.

You may generate a wide range of data visualizations without knowing how to code. With features like one-click regression analysis, which simplifies the curve, prism enables you to work more efficiently rather than more laboriously.

Benefits

- **Statistical analysis**: Regression analysis, survival analysis, regression analysis, t-tests, nonparametric comparisons, and more are all available in prism's extensive library of statistical studies. With the library of functions offered in plain language, you can skip statistical jargon and use a criteria checklist to make sure you've selected the right statistical test.
- **Collaboration:** Prism enables improved team collaboration because all project data is kept in a single, shareable file. By allowing others to follow your work step-by-step, you might gain new perspective and boost your team's overall research efforts.
- **Real-time updates:** The results and graphs are updated simultaneously in real time if any changes are made to data sets or analysis.

Statistical packages are used to:
- Investigate dataset information and showcase it.
- Investigate the connections between the data points.
- Analyze data to spot underlying trends and patterns.
- Create models of probability and assess their reliability.
- Utilize analytical algorithms to provide future predictions.
- Find practical insights.

INTRODUCTION TO MICROSOFT WORD

Word processing is the process of using a computer application to create, edit, and format text documents. One of the most advanced word processors on the market, Microsoft Word 2013 is a component of the Microsoft Office 2013 software suite. Word makes it simple and fast to generate a wide variety of professional and personal documents, from the most straightforward letter to the most intricate report. You can utilise Word's many desktop publishing tools to improve documents' appearances and make them easier to read and visually appealing.

The following uses for Microsoft Word are possible:
- To design business papers with a range of graphics, such as images, charts, and diagrams.
- To save and reuse pre-written text as well as structured elements like sidebars and cover pages.
- To design letterheads and letters for both personal and professional use.
- To create various documents, such as invitation cards or resumes, etc.
- To draught a variety of letters, from straightforward office memos to legal copy and reference materials.

How to Use Microsoft Word?

Assuming Microsoft Office 2010 is set up on your computer, follow these instructions to launch the Word programme.
Step 1 – Click the **Start** button.

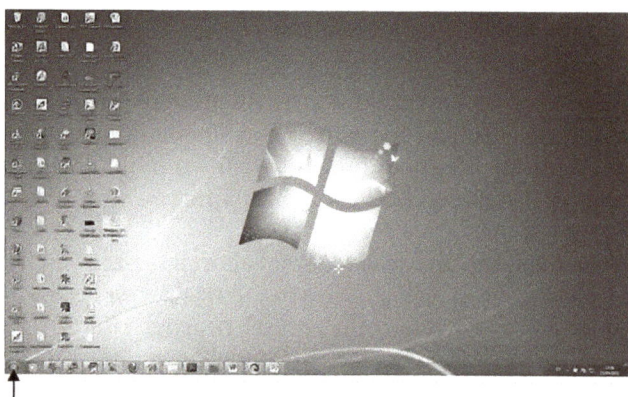

Start button

Introduction of Computer Application for Patient Care Delivery System and Nursing Practice

Step 2 – Click the **All Programs** option from the menu.

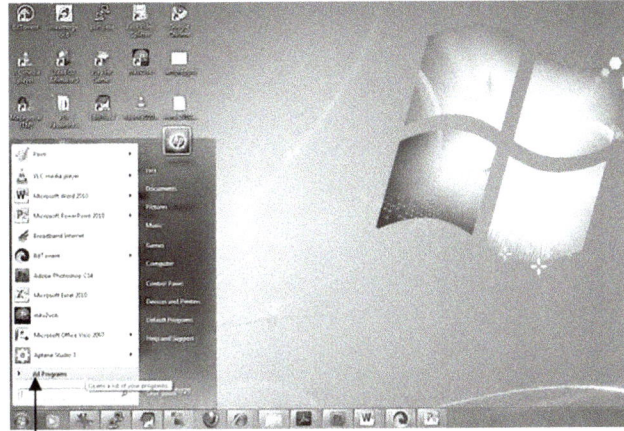

All programs

Step 3 – Search for **Microsoft Office** from the submenu and click it.

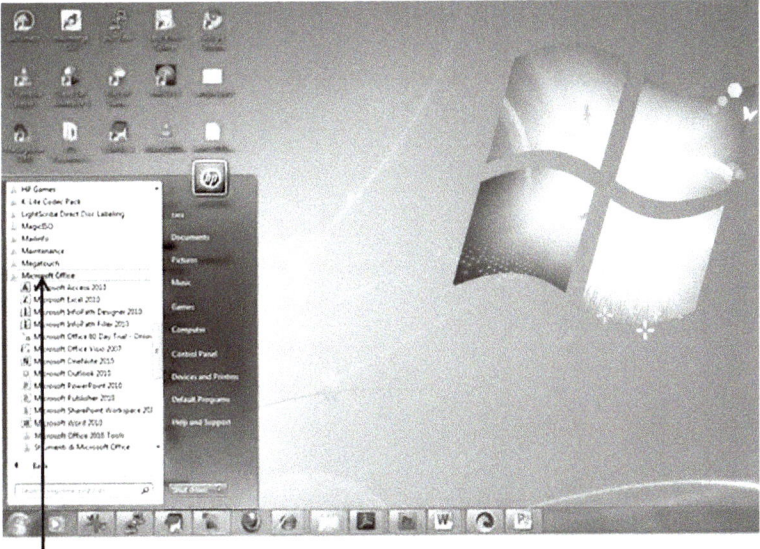

Microsoft office

Step 4 – Search for **Microsoft Word 2010** from the submenu and click it.

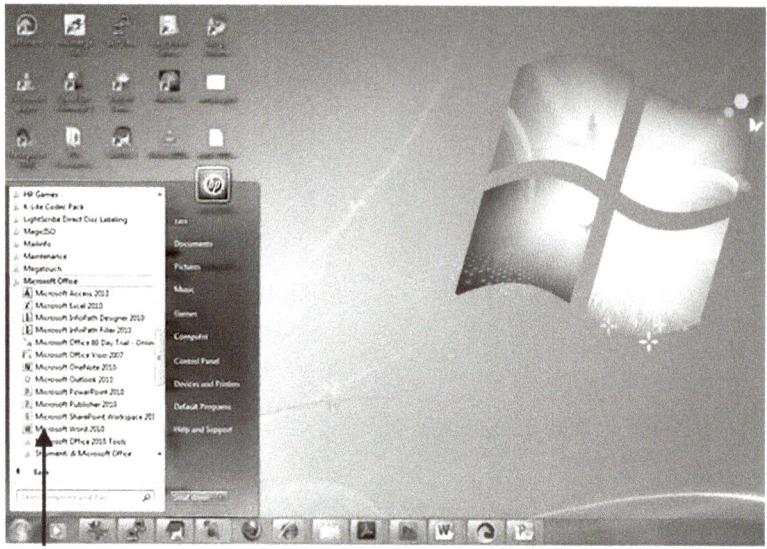

Microsoft Word 2010

This will launch the Microsoft Word 2010 application and you will see the following window.

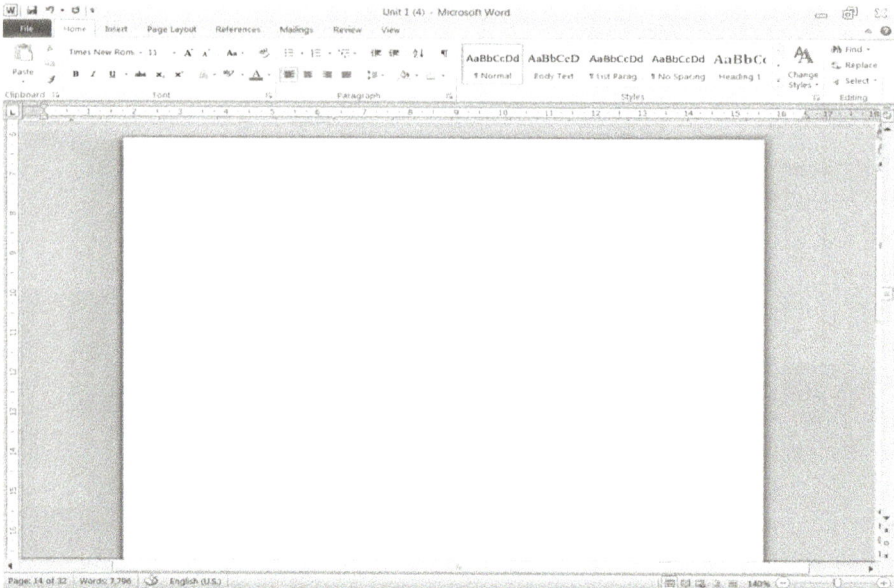

Introduction of Computer Application for Patient Care Delivery System and Nursing Practice

The initial window you see when you launch the Word application is shown below. Let's examine the numerous crucial components of this window.

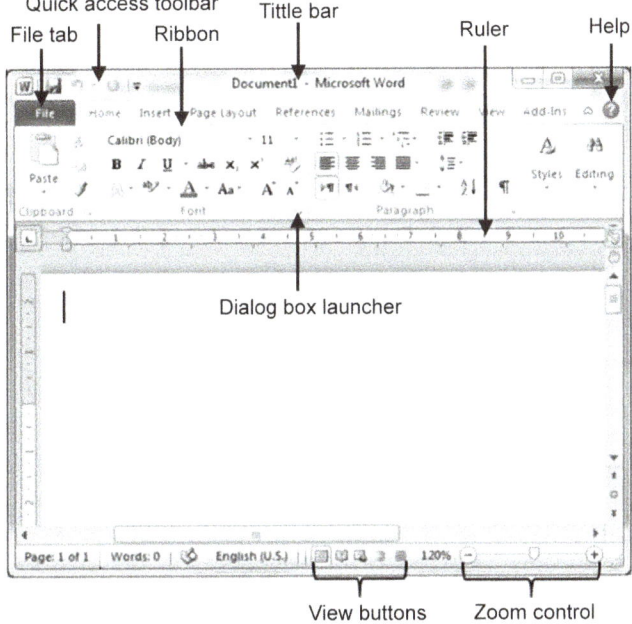

The Office button from Word 2007 has been replaced by the File tab. To access the Backstage view, click it. Here you can create new documents, open or save existing ones, print documents, and perform other tasks involving files.

Accessibility Toolbar

This is located immediately above the File tab. The most often used Word commands can conveniently rest here. This toolbar can be adjusted to your preferences.

Ribbon

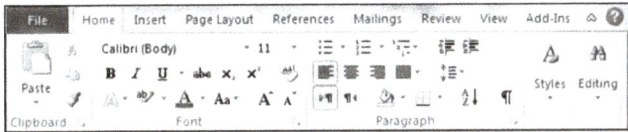

Commands on the ribbon are divided into three categories: First category is group, second is name, third is help.

Tabs are collections of linked instructions that show across the top of the Ribbon. The ribbon tabs Home, Insert, and Page Layout are a few examples.

Groups

They gather together relevant commands; on the Ribbon, each group's name may be found beneath the group. For instance, a collection of font-related commands or a group of alignment-related commands, etc.

Name Bar

This is located at the top of the window and in the centre. Program and document titles are displayed in the title bar.

A horizontal ruler and a vertical ruler are both included in Rulers Word. Setting margins and tab stops requires using the horizontal ruler, which is visible just below the Ribbon. To determine the vertical positioning of components on the page, utilise the vertical ruler, which is visible on the left edge of the Word window.

Help

The Aid You can use the icon at any moment to obtain assistance with words. This offers great tutorials on a variety of word-related topics.

Text Entry using Microsoft Word 2010

Let's talk about text entry using Microsoft Word 2010 in this chapter. Let's check out how simple adding text to a Word document is. We'll presume you're aware that Word launches with a brand-new document shown by default, as seen below.

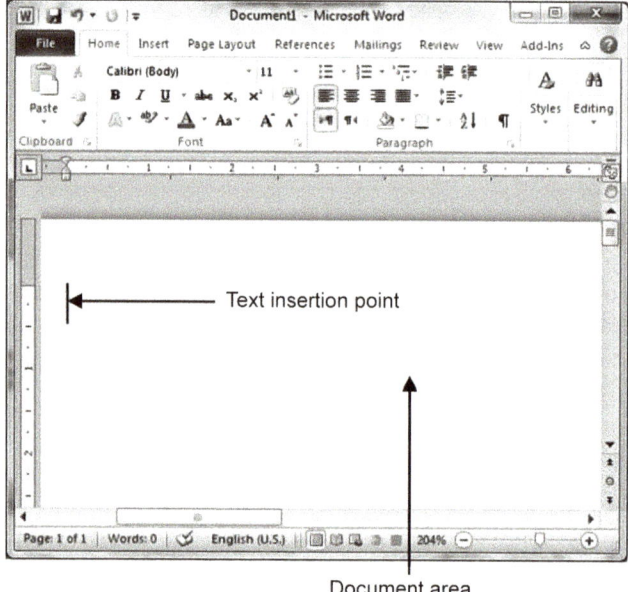

The text-entry area is called the document area. The insertion point, which is shown by the flashing vertical bar, indicates where the text will appear as you input. Keep the cursor where you want to insert the text and start typing. As illustrated here, we only typed the words "Hello Word" twice. As you enter, text appears to the left of the insertion point.

Introduction of Computer Application for Patient Care Delivery System and Nursing Practice

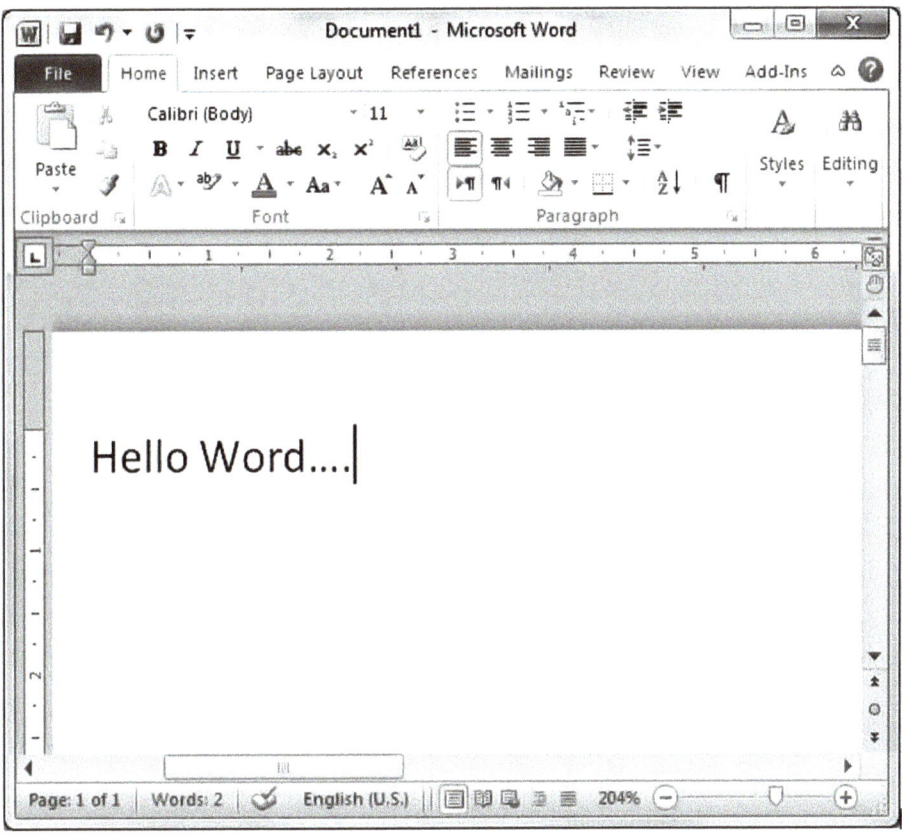

The two key ideas that will aid you in typing are as follows:

To begin a new line, you don't have to press Enter. Word begins a new line as soon as the insertion point reaches the end of the previous one. To add a new paragraph, you must press Enter.

Moving with Mouse

Use the Tab key rather than the spacebar to add more spaces between words. Utilizing proportional fonts will enable proper text alignment.

How to navigate Word 2010 will be covered in this chapter. Word offers a variety of keyboard and mouse navigation options for documents.

Simply click in your text anywhere on the screen to move the insertion place. There could be times when a document is so large that you are unable to see where you want to move. As seen in the following screenshot, you must use the scroll bars here.

Introduction of Computer Application for Patient Care Delivery System and Nursing Practice

Let's start by writing some sample text. There is a shortcut that can be used to create a sample text. Create a new document, enter =rand(), and then save it. The content listed below will be produced by Word for you.

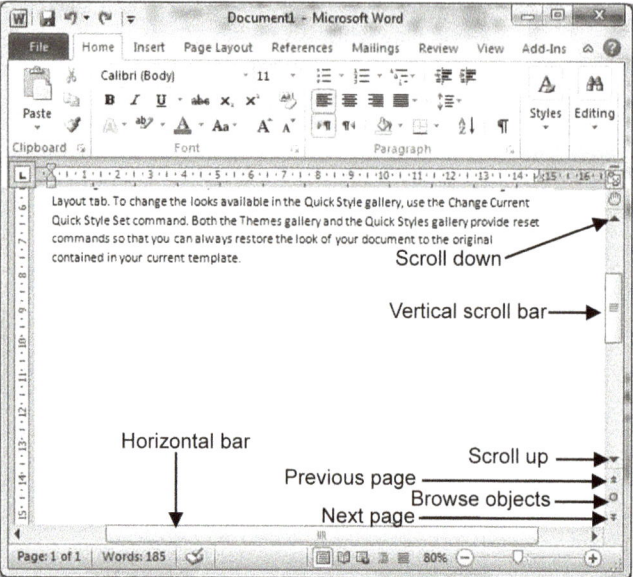

Moving with Keyboard

The insertion point is also moved by the keyboard commands listed below when you use them to navigate through your document:

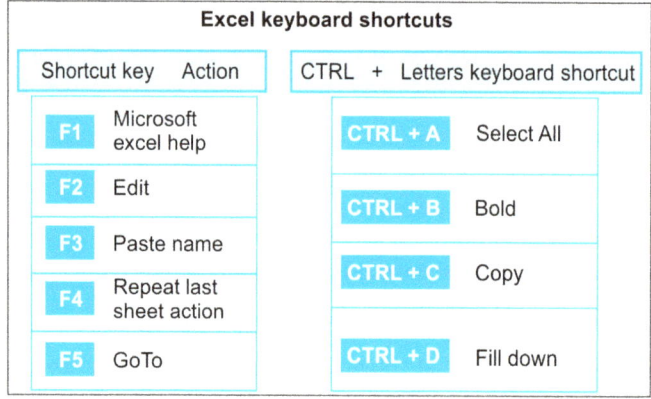

Introduction of Computer Application for Patient Care Delivery System and Nursing Practice

Saving New Document

It is time to save your new Word document once you have finished typing in it in order to protect your work from being lost. The steps to save a modified Word document are as follows:

Step 1 – **Click the** File tab **and select the** Save As **option.**

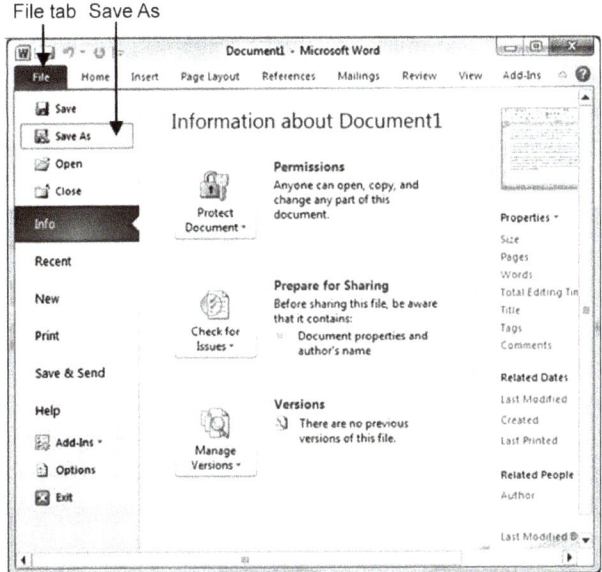

Step 2 – Select a folder where you will like to save the document, Enter the file name which you want to give to your document and Select the Save As **option, by default it is the** .docx **format.**

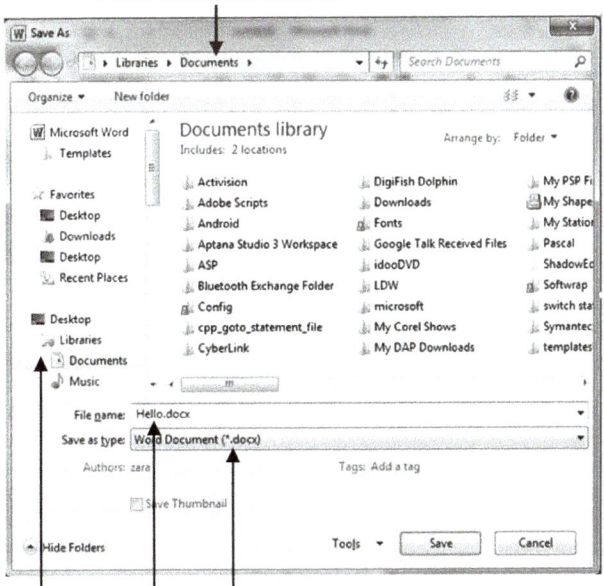

Step 3 – Finally, click on the Save **button and your document will be saved with the entered name in the selected folder.**

MICROSOFT EXCEL

Microsoft Excel 2000 is an application suite that runs on Windows. When entering, modifying, analyzing, and storing data, it is quite helpful. Operations on numerical data in arithmetic, like addition, with addition, subtraction, multiplication, and division. You can arrange the numbers and characters in some easy problems using the provided criteria (such as ascending, descending, etc.) formulae for finance, math, and statistics.

How to Open Microsoft Excel?

Running Excel is not different from running any other Windows program. If you are running Windows with a GUI like (Windows XP, Vista, and 7) follow the following steps:
- Click on start menu
- Point to all programs
- Point to Microsoft Excel
- Click on Microsoft Excel

EXCEL WORKSHEET

You can construct worksheets in Excel that function much like paper ledgers and even make computations automatically. Each workbook in an Excel file contains a number of worksheets. On the worksheet's top and left side are grey buttons that display the labels for the columns and rows, which are represented by letters and numbers. A cell is the point where a column and a row cross. The column letter and row number make up the cell address for each spreadsheet cell. Text, numbers, and mathematical formulas can all be contained in cells.

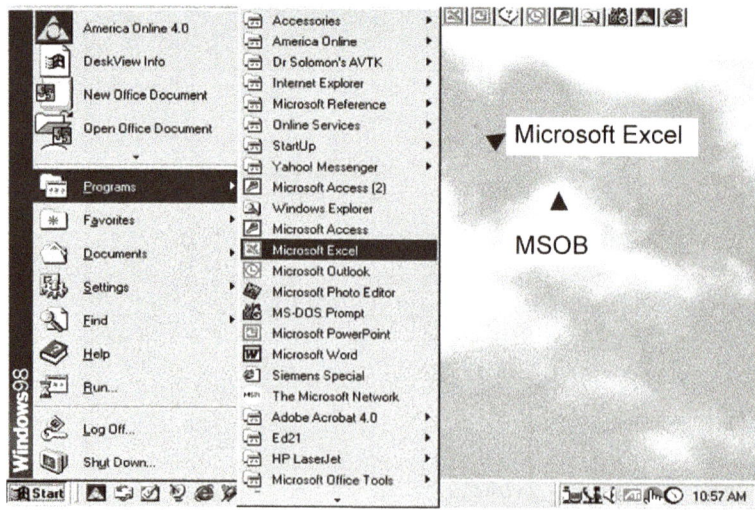

Introduction of Computer Application for Patient Care Delivery System and Nursing Practice

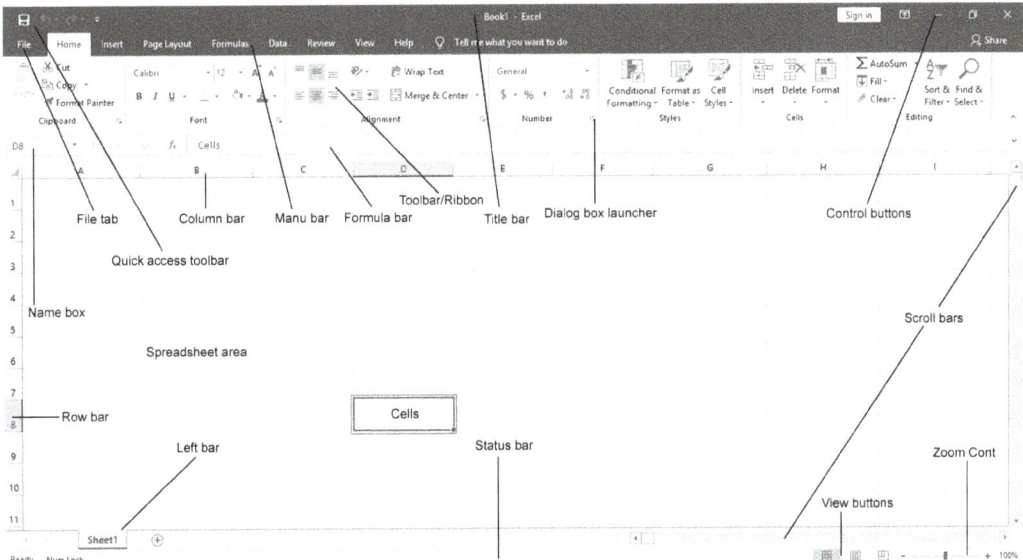

Standard Toolbar

You can rapidly access fundamental Excel commands from this toolbar at the top of the screen, immediately below the menu bar.

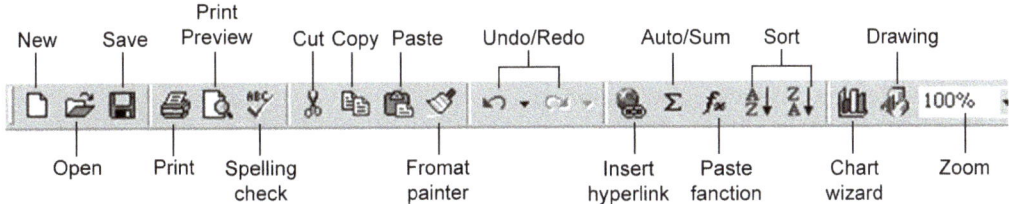

SELECTING CELLS AND RANGES

You must pick a cell or range before you can insert data into your worksheet. Cell A1 in an Excel worksheet is already selected as active. A worksheet cell that is active will appear to have a darker border than other worksheet cells. Using your mouse pointer to choose a cell is the easiest method. Drag the mouse pointer to the desired cell and use the right mouse button to select it. Anything you type is entered into the cell. Click on a cell, hold down the left mouse button, and then drag the mouse pointer to the final cell of the range you wish to pick to select a group of cells. For choosing cells, you can also use the keyboard shortcuts listed at the conclusion of this lesson.

Resizing Rows and Columns

There are two ways to resize rows and columns:
1. Drag the line beneath the label of the row you want to resize to change its size. By moving the line to the right of the label for the column you wish to resize, you can resize a column in a similar way.
2. To input a numerical number for the row's height or the column's width, click the row or column label and choose Format-Row-Height or Format-Column-Width from the menu bar.

EXCEL FEATURES

Excel offers a variety of functions that might help you with your assignment. Among the key characteristics are as follows:
- **AutoSum**: Aids in adding the contents of a group of related cells.
- **List AutoFill:** When a new item is added to the end of a list, cell formatting is automatically extended.
- The AutoFill tool enables you to swiftly fill cells with repetitive or sequential data, such as repeated text, numbers, or dates in chronological order.
- **AutoFill:** This feature also allows you to change numbers and text. You may design a variety of geometric forms, arrows, flowchart components, stars, and more using the 4 AutoShapes toolbar. You can create your own graphs using these shapes.
- **Wizard:** It helps you work successfully while you are working.
- **Charts:** You can give a graphical representation of your data using the tools for charts, which include pie, bar, line, and other charts.
- **PivotTable:** It lets you to execute data analysis and generate reports like recurring financial statements, statistical reports, etc. by quickly flipping and adding data. Graphical analysis of intricate data linkages is also an option.
- **Shortcut Menus:** By clicking the right mouse button, commands that are appropriate for the work you are performing show as shortcut menus.

MICROSOFT POWERPOINT

Getting Started

- The tool that helps you sell your message is PowerPoint. A presentation tool called PowerPoint is used to make transparencies for the overhead projector in addition to creating stunning slide shows with text, graphics, audio, and video.
- The Office 2007 programme that is the simplest to learn is PowerPoint. You can quickly produce attractive content for your sales pitch, lecture, or the screen in your storefront. Most of the work may be done for you via PowerPoint, allowing you to focus on crafting your messages effectively.
- Your machine won't have to work very hard to run PowerPoint. Therefore, considering your message's presentation will have a bigger impact on your results.

Ribbons and Tabs

- Like the other programmes in the Office suite, PowerPoint now has a fresh, modern style. The usual navigation bars and toolbars have been replaced with the new "Ribbon," which

Introduction of Computer Application for Patient Care Delivery System and Nursing Practice

is the first thing that stands out. The Ribbon has tabs, and each tab has buttons for the operations that were previously available in toolbars and menus. The Ribbon constantly adapts to the activity you are doing and is much more visually and task-oriented.
- The Ribbon takes some getting used to if you have spent a long time using toolbars and menus, but after sometime you grow used to it and even like it.

The Screen and its Elements

When you launch PowerPoint, a brand-new, empty presentation is already loaded. There is only one empty "slide" in the presentation. As opposed to Word, where we work with "pages," PowerPoint uses "slides." However, it is the same in practise.

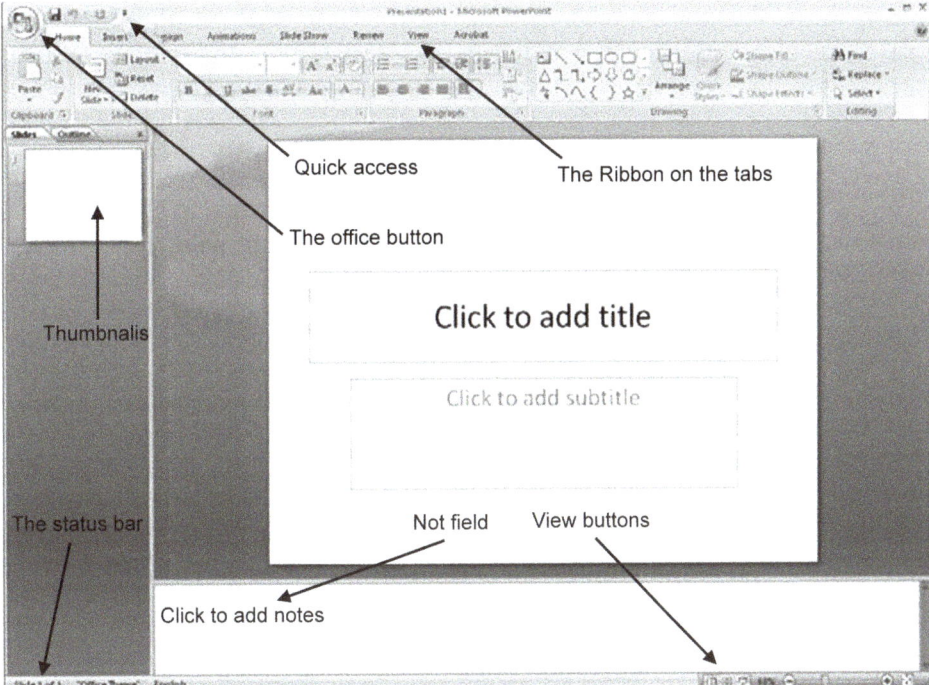

Basic Tasks in PowerPoint

There are a few processes you must always go through when creating a presentation. The following tasks must be performed before your presentation is ready, even though you presumably have an idea of what it should include.
- **Initial tasks**
  - Begin with an empty or contented template.
  - Change the slide format to print or screen show.
  - Pick a colour scheme and make any required adjustments.
- **Pour the content into the presentation**
  - On the top of the page, type a title.
  - Include slides with text, images, and graphs.

- **Polish the presentation**
  - Your slides' order should be adjusted.
  - If you are presenting a slide presentation on a screen, add transitions between slides.
  - If you're producing an on-screen show, add animations.
  - Test and make adjustments as needed.

SUMMARY

Excellent technical improvements have been bestowed upon the delivery of healthcare by science. The computerization of the entire healthcare delivery system is one such breakthrough. Computerization has made a significant contribution to the decline in medical errors and the issues they cause. The Electronic Medical Record (EMR) System, electronic prescriptions, personal digital assistants, computer automated cancer detection, and computerized theatre management applications are all examples of how healthcare is being delivered via computers. Another recent development is the use of voice recognition technologies in mobile healthcare settings. A specialization that combines computer science, information science, and nursing science to manage and share data, knowledge, and information to assist patients, nurses, and other clinicians in making decisions across all settings and roles. Prior to the turn of the new century, the computer was the most potent technical tool for changing the nursing profession. Nursing paper-based records have been converted to computer-based records thanks to the computer. The internet and computers are now necessary for the modern world to function on a large scale. Information technology (IT), computer systems, and its use in nursing information systems (NISs), nursing applications, and/or nursing informatics are all collectively referred to as "computers" (NI). "NI" has become a new word for these technologies that help nurses manage patient care and healthcare more effectively and efficiently while also increasing nurse accountability. Hospital nursing management has evolved as a result of the development of the computer that connects nursing departments. Computers are used to access and retrieve the majority of policy and procedure manuals. Also available online and either connected with the hospital's or the patient's EHR system, or in distinct nursing department systems, are workload measures, acuity systems, and other nursing department systems. At the bedside, nurses are using the Internet to access digital libraries, resources, and research procedures.

REVIEW QUESTION

1. Name four MS Excel programmes.
2. What are the key features of MS excel?
3. What makes a workbook different from a worksheet?
4. What kinds of information can be entered into worksheet cells?
5. Describe three different safeguards you use for your workbook.
6. What three methods are there for saving your workbook?
7. In a massive worksheet with hundreds of numbers and names, how do you locate the specific number or name you're looking for? Is it feasible to swap over a name or number for another one? How?
8. How do you choose a complete worksheet, a single column, a single row, a group of cells, or a single cell?

Introduction of Computer Application for Patient Care Delivery System and Nursing Practice

MULTIPLE CHOICE QUESTIONS

1. **The four common types of files are document files, presentation files, worksheet files and:**
   a. Software programmes
   b. Files in a database
   c. The system files
   d. Electronic records

2. **An application of voice and vision technology is in:**
   a. Database system
   b. Adobe photoshop database
   c. Video conferencing
   d. None of the above

3. **An electronic tool that allows information to be input, processed, and output is called _____.**
   a. Operating system
   b. Motherboard
   c. Personal computer
   d. CPU

4. **Name the brain of the computer that does the calculation, moving, and processing of information.**
   a. CPU
   b. RAM
   c. Motherboard
   d. Hard drive

5. **The "SPSS" is a package of programs for:**
   a. Manipulation
   b. Analyzing
   c. Presenting data
   d. All of these

6. **The "SPSS" is more widely use in:**
   a. Social and behavioral sciences
   b. Aerial science
   c. a and b
   d. None of these

7. **In SPSS online help is provides from the:**
   a. Help menu
   b. Context menu
   c. Help button
   d. All of these

8. **When SPSS is first open a default dialogue box appears that gives the user a number of:**
   a. Editing tutorial
   b. Date type
   c. Options
   d. a and b

9. **A source variables list is a list of variables from the _____ spreadsheet.**
   a. Data view
   b. Variable view
   c. a and b
   d. None of these

10. **SPSS stands for:**
    a. Statistical package for the social sciences
    b. Standard package for the social sciences
    c. a and b
    d. None of these

Answer Key

1. c
2. c
3. a
4. c
5. d
6. a
7. d
8. c
9. a
10. a

CHAPTER 2

Principles of Health Informatics

At the end of this chapter, student will able to learn about:
- Need of nursing informatics
- Objectives of nursing informatics
- Roles within nursing informatics
- Applications of nursing informatics
- Limitations of nursing informatics
- Theories of nursing informatics
- Use of data, information and knowledge in healthcare practice

TERMINOLOGIES

- **Health informatics:** To assist physicians in providing better healthcare, health informatics is the process of collecting, analysing, and managing health data as well as the use of medical theories in conjunction with health information technology systems.
- **Nursing informatics:** Nursing informatics includes all interactions between nurses and health IT systems. It manages patient records online and delegated the management of transitions of care to their nursing teams in their electronic health records.
- **Public health informatics:** The use of computer science, information, and technology in public health management, including disease surveillance, prevention, readiness, and health education.
- **Health information technology:** Medical practitioners and other healthcare organizations employ technological tools to collect, store, analyzes, retrieve, and share information.

INTRODUCTION

The field of technology has experienced a significant paradigm shift over the last few decades. Due to this paradigm change, the health care industry also became significantly more advanced and inventive. The technological revolution, particularly in the healthcare industry, has given nurses many chances to reduce responsibilities in clinical settings. For instance, preserving patient records on computers, inventories, medical supplies and equipment, and other tasks are

Principles of Health Informatics

now simple to complete. The area of nursing informatics today has more complex knowledge requirements and is a recognized specialization within the industry. Nursing informatics, which includes procedure and data, is seen as both a science and a system.

"Nursing informatics" refers to the application of computer science to the nursing profession and data processing.

NEED OF NURSING INFORMATICS

- Nursing informatics supports the decision-making of patients and nurses.
- Nursing informatics makes the clinical practice more effective by using nursing process.
- Nursing informatics can identify a need and demand for the nurses and healthcare settings.
- Nursing informatics helps in updating the knowledge and skills of nurses by proving continue nursing education to maintain competence and adheres to the overall education requirements of the profession.
- Nursing informatics defines the competencies for the area of specialty nursing practice.
- Nursing informatics provides mechanisms for supporting, reviewing, and disseminating research to support its knowledge base and evidence-based practice.
- Nursing informatics has defined educational criteria for specialty preparation in nursing.
- Has continuing education programs or other mechanisms for nurses in the specialty.

OBJECTIVES OF NURSING INFORMATICS

Nurse informatics has different roles and responsibilities in healthcare, each bringing value to the provision of patient care. Identified responsibilities of nursing informatics (HIMSS, 2012) include:
- Examine both financial and clinical data
- Promote the delivery of evidence-based, high-quality healthcare
- Present nursing information in standardized languages
- Enhance care continuity
- Support and make it easier to find resources and references
- Strengthen connections between medical professionals and patients
- Encourage cost-cutting measures and productivity targets
- Restructure the clinical workflow
- Support the management of change
- Use technology to maintain nursing job processes
- Encourage real multidisciplinary treatment

APPLICATIONS OF NURSING INFORMATICS

- **As a nursing practice:** Following are the application of nursing informatics in nursing practice.

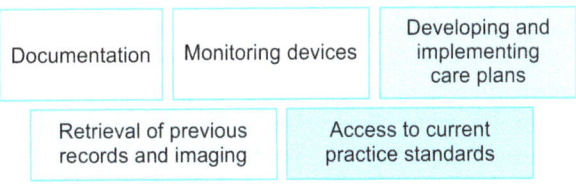

- **Nursing administration:** Following are the application of nursing informatics in nursing administration:

  - In staff scheduling systems
  - In cost and budget analysis
  - Monitoring of trends with quality and satisfaction data

- **Research:** Access to electronic databases like EBSCO, SCOPUS, and PubMed, as well as the internet, offers a wealth of resources for gathering information and doing research.
- **Education:** By using simulation, e-learning, teleconferencing, and software that is available for educational presentations and programmes, nursing informatics can be used to enhance the nursing education system.
- **Shareable knowledge:** Medical professionals gain a better understanding of diseases and efficient therapies by reading and comprehending the information in healthcare data. Then, suppliers can more easily exchange this information.
- **Patient education:** Health informatics provides additional information to healthcare organizations and clinicians, which may subsequently be disseminated to patients and the general public. Evidence-based instruction can lower the risk of injury and aid in disease prevention.
- **Patient involvement:** By converting patient records from hard copies.

LIMITATIONS OF NURSING INFORMATICS

- **Chances of losing data:** There could be issues with the computer losing data, more vulnerability to have viruses on the computer, which requires more time for the health workers to type in data.
- **Less physical interaction with students:** Informatics makes the teacher nurse to take lectures through online mode that will minimize the physical interaction with students. The best example is during lockdown period the education system faced many issues to deliver lectures that interfere with the understanding capacity of students.
- **Less interaction with patient:** Informatics system creates a less personal interaction with the patient and doctor, pertaining to their visit.
- **Time consuming:** Health informatics needs time to adapt in the era, where people used to keep records and reports on hard copies. It needs learning skills which is time taken process especially to people who shifted from 60s to modern era.
- **Over dependency:** Informatics makes the nurses dependent on technology. During the downtime system, it would be difficult to manage the patient data.
- **Lack of confidentiality:** Informatics system is more susceptible to network hackers. Which question on confidentiality of patient data.

THEORIES OF NURSING INFORMATICS

Theories in nursing informatics provides a framework and foundation which include concepts, network and relationships that assist in providing a complete structure of curriculum.
- **Systems theory:** Systems theory looks at interacting parts within boundaries, and can be seen with the use of technology and the body systems of patients.

- **Cognitive theory:** Cognitive theory can be related to input, output, and processing.
- **Change theory:** Change theory is applied in looking at the dynamic processes that are incorporated with nursing informatics.

USE OF DATA, INFORMATION AND KNOWLEDGE IN HEALTHCARE PRACTICE

The use of information and knowledge in healthcare can be categorized into four main streams such as:

1. **Health and education:** In the digital age, people can quickly find, access, learn from, and communicate with others. Education is now open, available, and accessible to everyone. Public awareness of communicable diseases, health status, preventative measures, and different modern diagnostic and treatment techniques is fostered via health education. This provides consumers the option to select the top medical facilities and practitioners to turn to for care so they can live a healthy life.
2. **Hospital management system:** Hospital management to successfully guide the organization. This aids management in overcoming the difficulties the hospital is now experiencing. It aids management in enhancing patient security and satisfaction, staying current with cutting-edge technology, being knowledgeable about population health and statistics, and staying on top of legislative mandates. The workplace can be strengthened in first place.
3. **Healthcare research:** Healthcare research aids in identifying potential disease eradication and disease reduction strategies. New technologies in diagnosis can speed up the process and cut costs. This provides therapy in advance, saving the lives of numerous people. The existing healthcare systems can be abolished and new models for efficient, high-quality treatment can be created through knowledge and information.
4. **Health data management:** Electronic medical data storage is the primary application of knowledge and information in hospitals. This makes it easier to access the information. Data can be provided to the patient or to the doctors for consultation thanks to knowledge and information. The patient can access their own medical records at anytime and anyplace.

Applied Examples of Knowledge and Information in Healthcare

- **Nanotechnology:** Nanotechnology is slowly but steadily making its way toward contributing to the medical sector of our country. Scientists have developed Nanobots that are capable of unclogging arteries and preventing the cases of heart attacks. Researchers are in the process of developing nanoparticles that will be able to cure neurological disorders in a better way. Nanotechnology is an area that has a lot of scope for further providing neck-breaking technology in this field.
- **Artificial intelligence:** It is no secret that humans as a species are the most intelligent and analytical on this planet. We are superior to any other organism when it comes to processing data in a logical and systematic matter. The only limitation we face is in terms of the amount of information we can process over a given amount of time. That is where the importance of Artificial Intelligence (AI) can be seen. Some of the applications of AI in healthcare are treatment design, virtual nurses, drug creation, health monitoring.
- **Real time data:** We are living in a world where every news and information comes to us 'live'. In today's day and age where everything is real time, many start-ups have come in the healthcare sector that are focusing on providing live status of your appointments on

your phone, queue management for hospitals/clinics, urgent online bookings in case of emergencies, door-to-door delivery of medicines, medical reports on your phone straight from the lab, etc. This has made a lot of people's life easier than it used to be before. In addition to this, it also saves up a lot of time.

Robotics: Advantage of having technology is that it makes our life much more efficient and easy. The entering of robotics in healthcare sector is one of the most advance move that humans have initiated in terms of medicine. There are robotic surgeries these days that are performed without the presence of a physician. Robotic assistance is also there at some places where robots help in medical equipment and telehealth. They also help in monitoring procedures. Robots are also performing surgeries these days in delicate areas of our body, such as human brain, etc.

- **Virtual reality:** Virtual reality in the healthcare sector have made significant developments in conditions, such as autism, lazy eye, chronic pain, etc. A lot of people associate virtual reality only with cinema but virtual reality has a lot more applications than that. Many labs use virtual reality to treat chronic pain. Virtual reality is also used for speedy recovery from fatal brain injuries. It also helps in medical education as a lot of institutes use it to give students live experience by streaming surgical operations, etc. This revolutionary solution is safe and affordable at the same time.

SUMMARY

Information science, computer science, and healthcare come together in health informatics. The tools, systems, and techniques needed to acquire, store, retrieve, and utilize information in health and biomedicine efficiently are the focus of this discipline. The field of health informatics is diverse and developing. The healthcare sector's emphasis on evidence-based medicine, quality improvement, and patient data protection and accessibility is driving demand. HI is evolving to keep up with advances in big data, data security regulations, and artificial intelligence. Standards for computing power, data processing, and data security are developing and getting better. The future of health informatics will continue to grow through technological and standards advances, the acceptance of patient information rights, and the modernization of healthcare, which is now well under way.

REVIEW QUESTION

1. Define health informatics and need of health informatics in nursing practices.
2. Explain the applications of health informatics in nursing.
3. What are the limitations of nursing informatics?
4. Explain the use of data information system in healthcare setting.

MULTIPLE CHOICE QUESTIONS

1. EMR is an abbreviation for which of the following?
    a. Electronic Medical Record
    b. Emergency Medical Record
    c. E-Medical Resource
    d. Electronic Medical of Recording
2. Which of the following is a feature of the EHR?
    a. Personal family record
    b. Continuity of care record
    c. Application provider
    d. Personal record

Principles of Health Informatics

3. **Why did healthcare providers perceive EHR systems to lack safety?**
   a. Data hacking
   b. Because of possible power outages
   c. Because of possible computer "crashes"
   d. All of these

4. **All of the following are benefits of implementing EHRs, *except*:**
   a. At the point of care for a patient, access to their medical records is possible.
   b. Past medical histories and family medical histories can be simply shared with the healthcare provider.
   c. EHRs are more time-consuming than paper charts.
   d. It is simple to educate and view the healthcare provider's immunization records.

5. **Which of the following can be eliminated with the use of EHRs?**
   a. Nurses
   b. Clerical staff
   c. Hanwritten notes, orders, and prescriptions
   d. All of these

6. **What is one benefit of an EHR over paper charts?**
   a. EHR is centralized.
   b. EHR can become cluttered.
   c. Paper charts are always more accessible than EHR charts.
   d. EHR cannot be accessed off site.

7. **Which of the following describes a method in which EHRs enhance communication between providers and their staff?**
   a. Instant messaging
   b. SMS
   c. Digital vocabulary
   d. Voice recognition

8. **EHR is an acronym for:**
   a. Emergency health record
   b. Electronic health record
   c. Emergency health repository
   d. Electronic health repository

9. **Which of the following may increase the price of EHR implementation?**
   a. Computer hardware
   b. Staff training
   c. System maintenance
   d. All of these

10. **In what ways do EHR provide meaningful improvements with the use of e-prescribing?**
    a. Cost
    b. Quality
    c. Patient safety
    d. All of these

Answer Key

1. a   2. b   3. d   4. c   5. c
6. a   7. a   8. b   9. d   10. d

CHAPTER 3

Information System in Healthcare

At the end of this chapter, student will able to learn about:
- Roles of information system in healthcare industry
- Structure and architect of healthcare information system
- Hospital Information System
- Components of hospital information system
- Importance of hospital information system for beneficiaries
- Types of hospital information systems

TERMINOLOGIES

- **ADT (patient administration) interface:** ADT stands for "admissions, discharges, and transfers" and is a digital method that exchanges patient registration information (e.g. demographics) between two systems.
- **Cerner:** A company that specializes in electronic medical record software out of kansas city, missouri, offering software solutions across the globe.
- **Discrete results:** Results that are broken down into their individual values, units and reference ranges. These results can be more easily tracked and charted.
- **Data extraction (or abstraction):** A process by which information on documents (structured or unstructured) is saved off in another format that can be then used for other purposes.
- **Document management system (DMS):** An internal computer system within the organization that is the repository for patient documents. The documents are generally organized so that the documents can be found in a patient's electronic medical record.
- **Electronic medical record (EMR):** The digital collection of a patient's medical data in one provider's office, (i.e. hospital, clinic...etc.) that can be shared across different healthcare settings.
- **Electronic medical record software:** The piece of software that collects, stores and allows for the viewing of the patient's medical data. Examples include epic and cerner.
- **Health information management (HIM):** The part of the hospital organization responsible for the management of digital and hard-copy information that is important for providing patient care.

- **Informatics (clinical informatics):** The study of information technology within healthcare conducted by and for clinicians. Clinical informaticians transform healthcare by analyzing, designing, implementing, and evaluating information and communication systems that enhance individual and population health outcomes, improve [patient] care, and strengthen the clinician-patient relationship.

ROLE AND ARCHITECTURE OF INFORMATION SYSTEMS

Introduction

Our society's healthcare system is essential. Recently, the way that people think about healthcare has changed dramatically, raising expectations and driving up demand for high-quality medical services and facilities. People can get medical help from hospitals. All sizes of healthcare businesses must manage and integrate clinical, financial, and operational information. A hospital information system needs to be established in order to complete this duty.

Every industry has undergone evolution as a result of technological development, which has sped up and smoothed the management process while benefiting more people globally. Healthcare is not an exception. Technology has greatly aided the fields of business, information technology, healthcare informatics, and healthcare data.

The health information system (HIS) is a technological marvel for the healthcare sector that makes managing patient data incredibly efficient. The adoption of this system contributes to a higher standard of patient care, lower operating costs, error-free administration data, and a more organized internal management process.

Definition

A common word used to describe electronic systems created to manage healthcare data is healthcare information systems, also known as "HIS." Systems that gather, maintain, transmit, and store patient records fall under this category.

HCISs as powerful ICT-based tools able to make healthcare delivery more effective and efficient. —*Rodrigues (2010)*

In order to collect and manage all the data linked to both clinical and administrative procedures, healthcare organizations, doctors, patients, and policy makers depend on HCISs, which are made up of a variety of applications.

Role of Information System in Healthcare

Organized and Coordinated Treatment Process

Protected health information (PHI) sharing between businesses and service providers is made incredibly simple thanks to the Health Information Approach, a technology-driven system. Patients can receive seamless and coordinated care from healthcare providers as a result of this approach.

Improved Patient Safety

With the aid of health information systems, one may save all the information and share it across many databases to increase patient safety because it facilitates easy access to patient data. Every time there are any problems involving the health of the patients, it sends an alarm signal. For instance, programme security checks can send alerts to healthcare providers about potentially harmful side effects of a patient using a medication without a prescription. By doing this, any severe error that results from a lack of information being available when making decisions can be avoided.

Betterment in Patient Care

By collecting and storing patient information, such as diagnosis reports, medical histories, allergic reactions, vaccination records, treatment information plans, test results, etc., health information systems provide healthcare professionals with a comprehensive and organized framework that enables them to interact with their patients in a better way and ultimately provide care to them more effectively.

Process of Performance Analysis without Hassles

Health information systems can be used in a variety of ways to evaluate staff performance, analyze patient care, and gauge an organization's effectiveness and stability. By converting all records to computers, HIS reduces paperwork. Any staff-related decision can be based on a person's skill set and after paying close attention to the particulars of past performance.

Transformation in Clinical Procedure

HIS aids in handling any stressful conditions that patients may encounter. You may virtually observe the movement of patients and what each individual patient goes through when they interact with medical professionals, office staff, lab technicians, and financial assistance. Paying close attention to this assists in identifying the areas that can use improvement.

Avoiding of Medical Errors

Health information systems provide accurate reports and information since they maintain less paper work and automate and computerize processes. Various drug errors can be prevented as a result, and patients' safety can be guaranteed.

Easy Accessibility to Patients' Information

According to a report released by the World Health Organization, the Health Information System collects data from the healthcare sector and other relevant industries, analyzes the data to ensure its overall quality, relevance, and timeliness, and then converts the data into information for health-related decision-making (WHO). Additionally, the more reliable the information, the better chance you have to make a choice, implement any policy or law, carry out health research, put any programme for training and development into action, and oversee the delivery of services, as well as after paying attention to details of prior performance.

Cost Effective

Information systems for health enable health organizations to allocate resources strategically and potentially save significant sums of money, energy, and resources. As a result, it is possible to improve healthcare services for patients while significantly reducing costs.

Time Management

Health information systems not only aid with financial savings but also time savings. HIS saves a substantial amount of time in the coordination of patient care and smooth hospital management by automating all patient personal actions and computerizing all patient information.

Improved Patient Satisfaction

Health information systems boost patient happiness by adding value to the therapeutic process, which also makes the daily work of healthcare administrators and professionals easier. Patients can rely on the services, and when an organization gains a solid reputation with in healthcare industry, more patients are drawn to it, and it experiences a significant return on investment.

After examining the capabilities of HIS, it is clear that HIS offers healthcare professionals a wide range of possibilities to provide patients with better treatment while reducing costs and streamlining processes.

Architectural Models for Healthcare Information Systems

Health information systems (HISs) are essential to the delivery of healthcare and the collection of payment for it. Healthcare providers encounter numerous issues with their HISs as a result of poor building design.

From a functional viewpoint, an HCIS supports three main levels of a healthcare system:
- **Central government at national and regional level:** Central planning, resource management, setting of policies and procedures to be followed, general controls over financial performance, and quality and safety monitoring are all examples of central government at the national and regional levels. This level is organized differently depending on the type of each country's healthcare system, whose fundamental paradigms can be either the mutual-private model typical of the United States or the Anglo-Saxon model.
- **Primary care health services:** This level includes all of the infrastructure necessary to facilitate the delivery of services to the populace of a country or region. All service providers are included, including neighbourhood practises, general practitioners, etc.
- **Secondary care health services:** This level largely refers to the mechanisms that facilitate communication between healthcare professionals. Architecture of information system in hospital.

An optimal local area network (LAN) architecture for a single hospital is one with a multi-tiered client-server structure. Users enter and retrieve data using clients, which are computers equipped with display monitors and data entry devices such keyboards and mouse, and subsequently store the information via the storage server into storage devices (hard disks). All of the layers are connected by a network of cables that are joined by switches and routers. Wireless elements might also be present in the network. An example of a typical HIS system architecture implementation is shown below.

Typical HIS System Architecture

The architecture plan of hospital needs some of the physical layout which are as follows:
- Adequate processing speed
- A sufficient amount of ram to temporarily store data, while it is being viewed or typed.
- A monitor with a display that can show both data and apps.
- Data entry devices, such as keyboard, bar-code reader, image scanner, and pointing devices like a mouse.
- An OS front interface that enables the operation of the aforementioned hardware and makes it easier to communicate with the server places that use complicated visuals should have video/graphic cards.

Hospital Information System Hybrid

Clients typically choose desktop and laptop/tablet PCs with powerful CPUs and lots of memory. Through the use of appropriate cables and wireless connections, they are connected to the network. These can be used as hybrid clients or both thick and thin clients.
- **Thick hybrid:** Client PCs with quick CPUs and lots of RAM memory are needed for a thick client installation. Applications software is either fully or partially installed on them.

☐ **Thin hybrid:** In a thin client strategy, only a browser is loaded into the client. When necessary, the applications are obtained from the applications server.

Less RAM memory is needed and lower end CPUs may be utilized. However, because images and graphs must be presented in an HIS setup, the thin client hardware—low end computers with little computing power and memory—is insufficient. PCs are more suited in their place. Each client can be used as an image viewer as well as for a wide range of administrative and medical (office automation, e-mail) applications. All of these applications must be supported by the operating system (OS) for the front end (presentation logic). Additionally, it ought to support user interfaces (GUIs) that meet users' needs.

Web Network

In the local area network, the system might use web technologies. Similar to thin clients, a web client can be used to host the browser. A secure network, such as a Virtual Private Network (VPN). SERVERS, should be used to connect to the hospital's LAN if a care provider needs access to HIS through patients in locations other than the hospital, such as from home or another hospital/clinic.

The server-storage system in a thorough integrated HIS must support both management applications and patient care applications. A hospital operates every day of the year, 365 days a year, hence the system shouldn't malfunction. Currently, a 99.9 percent uptime level is desired. The ability to make apps available and guarantee that data can be saved and retrieved without interruption should be duplicated in order to accomplish this. This translates into offering multiple locations for each application to dwell and store data.

Redundancy is the ability of the system to continue operating even if a component fails. There are many users of the system in patient care at any given moment, which generates a lot of data flow. Application servers and database servers both need to have enough processing power and memory to handle requests. A lot of data is typically needed at any given time, and it builds up over time. The storage device must be able to accept and release data quickly and have a big storage capacity.

A full system must support other functions in addition to daily operations. Therefore, copies of systems and applications must be made available for other crucial purposes. Domains are the alternative forms of clinical applications and distinct databases. These often consist of:

☐ **Production or operations domain:** The operations domain provides real-time, accurate data for daily use.
☐ **Analytical domain:** Reports can be produced by analyzing actual data, though not necessarily real-time data.
☐ The build or test domain contains a version of the programmes that is frequently distinct from that of the operational environment. It might have false information in it.
☐ **Train domain:** The train domain uses the same software as the operations domain, but it only uses made-up or fictitious data.

Despite the variety of domains and versions, this does not always imply the need for separate server-storage hardware.

Application Server

Managerial applications and clinical apps typically employ different servers and storage systems. This may necessitate the installation of numerous physical servers and storage systems in addition to the requirement for duplication. The number of physical servers can be decreased by using virtualization technologies. It is possible to employ a cluster of physical servers (at least two). Many virtual servers will be housed on each physical server.

Information System in Healthcare

Users are able to communicate with servers and request help with the operation of an application or a specific feature, as well as with the entry or retrieval of data. Through the usage of the application server, the user may have access to any programmes that they choose (s). When the client approach is used, all of the application software is stored on the server that manages the applications. In the event that personal computers (PCs) are used, it is possible that the client computer will save part of the data. If the thin client technique is employed, the applications server houses all of the applications software. If PCs are used, some of the data might be stored on the client computer.

Database and Data Storage Hardware

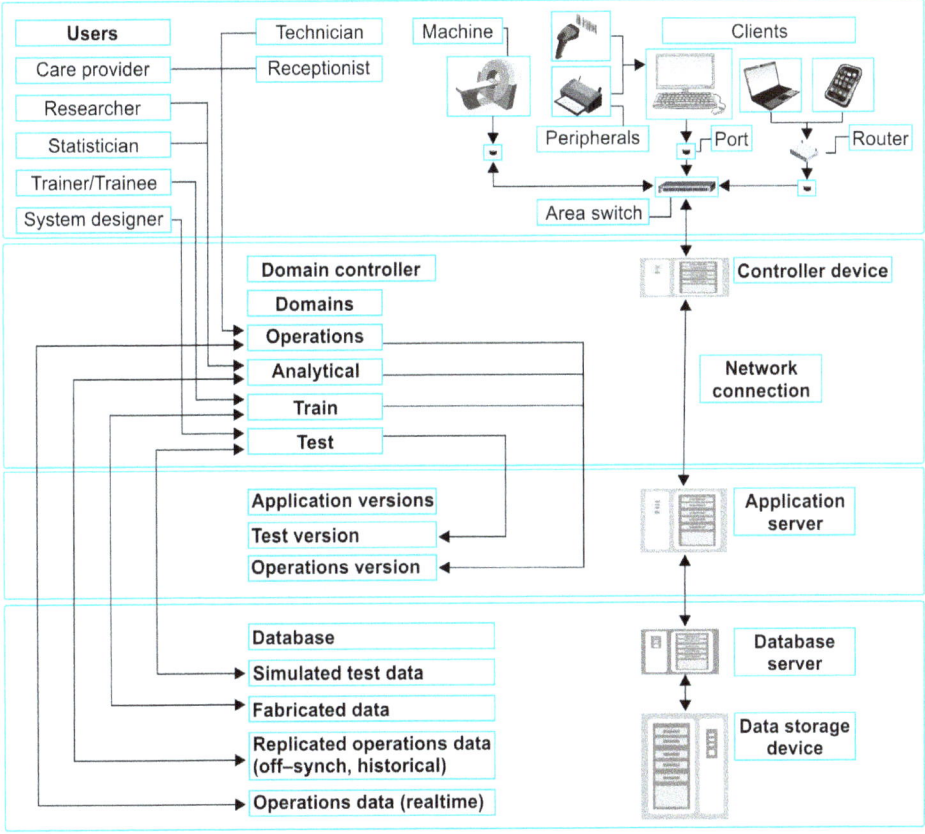

Fig. 3.1: Database domain.

Database Server

Data input and output from storage devices, such as storage area network (SAN storage) or network area storage are controlled by database servers or database/storage servers (NAS). The database management system is the programme that specifies the database's content and organizational structure (DBMS). Depending on the kind, it could be relational, hierarchical, or object-oriented. A suitable system software is required for both the database server and the DBMS (OS).

Information System in Healthcare

Currently, a set of hard drives serve as the data storage medium (disk array). Data backups are mostly stored on magnetic tapes (tape libraries). The network must possess the following characteristics:

- Sufficient bandwidth corresponding to volume of data that will traverse through two points to be connected.
- Redundancy to ensure an alternative passage of data if one route is impassible.

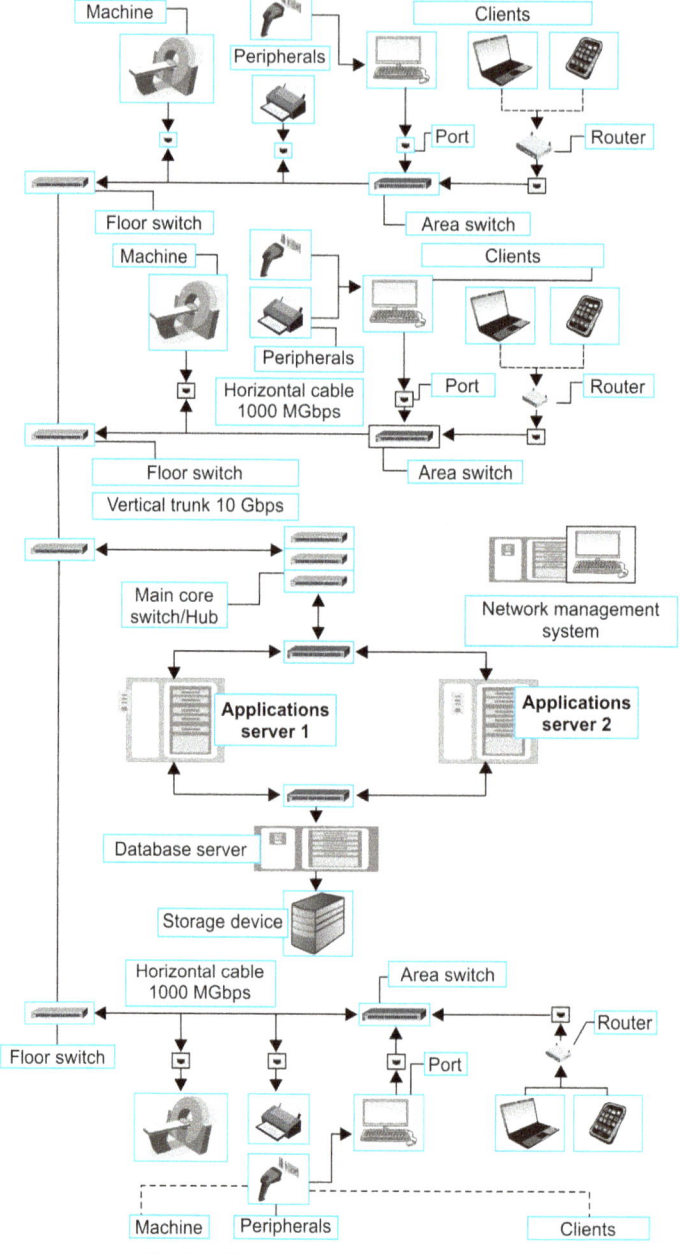

Fig. 3.2: Database management system.

Information System in Healthcare

One approach is to install two single mode fibre optic cables as the hospital's backbone, one on each side. Each cable's structure and diameter, which is typically 9/125 micrometres, influence the band-width, or rate at which data is transmitted, which is expressed in terms of bits per second (or other units of data per unit of time). Standard core cables can deliver data at a rate of 10 Gigabits per second. At the access level, the backbone is expanded using multimode cables made of four-core (50/125 micrometre) cables that can transmit data at speeds of 10, 100, and 1000 megabits per second.

Network Architecture

The domain controller (DC) allows the user to access the appropriate "domain" or version of the application or database, i.e., production or operations domain, analytical domain, build or test domain, train domain, in the HIS system as detailed here.

Phases to Use Network Domain

Phase 1: Privileges are set in order to determine who has access to a domain. The controller confirms the user's identity (by username and password). The active directory is the key component of the controller if the Microsoft Windows operating system is used.

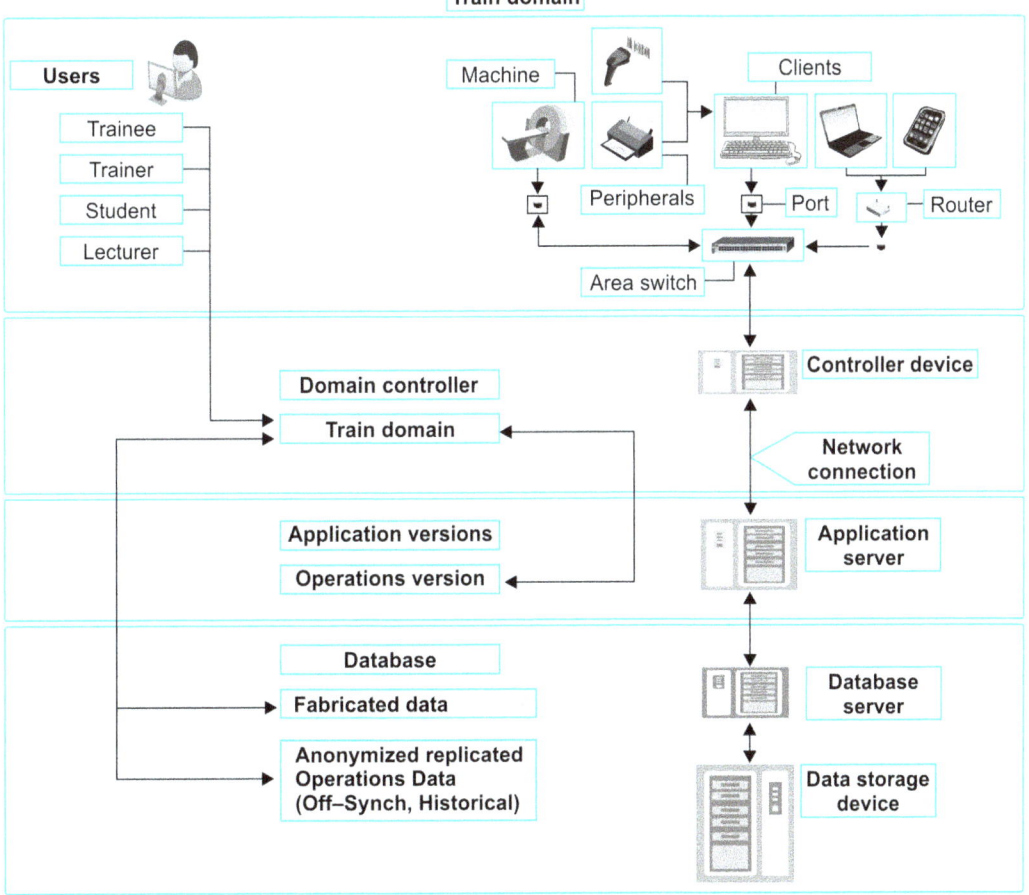

Fig. 3.3: Training domain database.

Phase 2: Users are granted access to the domain that matches the type of work they will be doing. For instance, the system should be configured so that users are forwarded to the train domain during training.

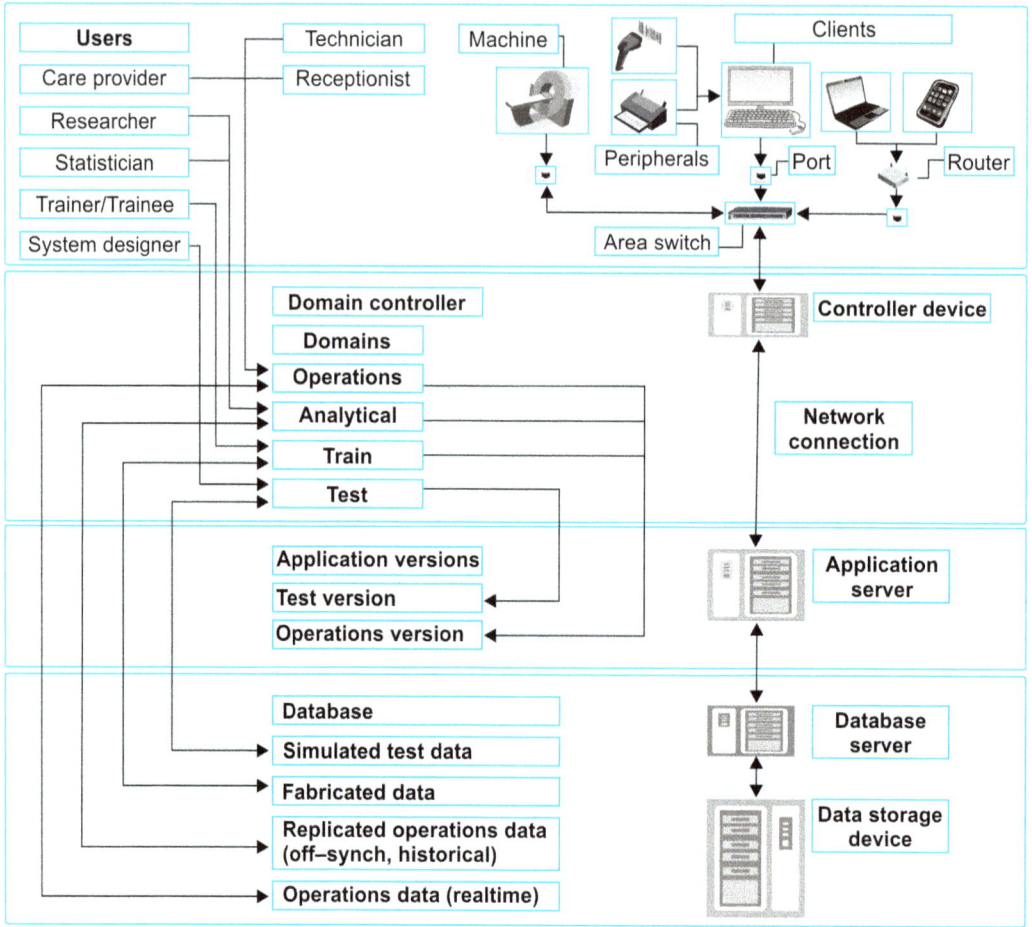

Fig. 3.4: Phase 2 : Train domain

Phase 3: The user employs the analytical domain when performing data analysis on historical data. (This section needs editing) at its core, active directory is a database management system. This database can be replicated using a multi-master replication technique over any number of server computers (referred to as domain controllers), allowing changes to be made to any independent copy while simultaneously propagating those changes to all other copies.

Phase 4: An enterprise's active directory database can be divided up into replication units called "Domains." The method of replication between server computers can be set up very flexibly to allow replication even in the event that communication between domain controller computers fails, as well as to replicate effectively between locations that might be connected via WAN connectivity with limited bandwidth. The active directory is used by windows as a repository for configuration data.

Phase 5: The most important of these purposes is the storage of user logon credentials (usernames and password hashes), so that computers can be set up to make use of this database and provide centralized single sign-on for many devices (referred to as "members" of the "Domain"). The explicit naming of user accounts from the active directory domain in permissions called access control lists (ACLs) or the logical grouping of user accounts into security groups are two ways to control access permissions to resources hosted by servers that are members of an active directory domain.

Phase 6: The active directory is where the names and memberships of these security groups are stored. The domain controller would act as a bridge between the front end and the server, whether it were located on a standalone computer or inside the primary server.

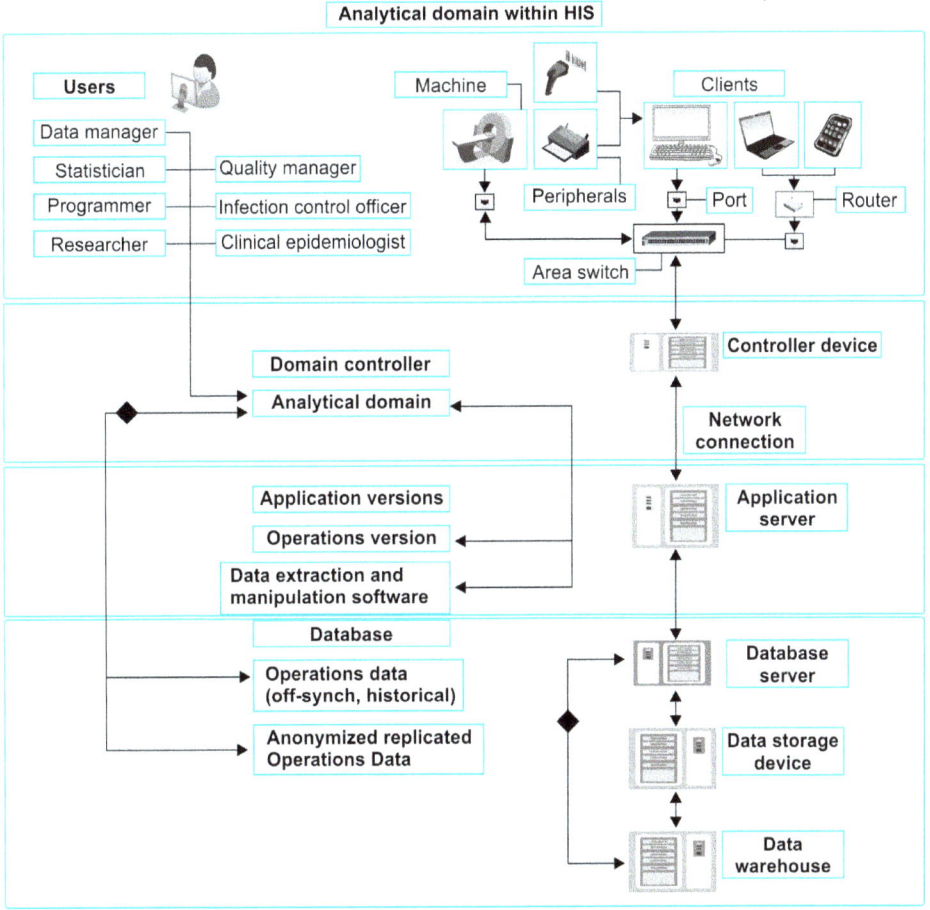

Fig. 3.5: Phase 3: Analytical domain.

System Manager

A domain is only set up for IT administration needs. Data on HIS patients is not accessible. Using a suite of network management systems made up of Network Configuration Manager, Storage Manager, Virtualization Manager, etc. (for example, solar winds or manage engine), access to sensitive information will be strictly controlled, including configurations of various devices in (servers, applications, network devices, storage devices), access credentials, SNMP settings, and access control lists. In accordance with a person's work category and status, privilege will be divided. Our change management software supports compliance with laws like HIPAA and PCI by using system administrator staff roles, permissions, and activity tracking available in the same application to guard against illegal network configuration modifications.

> **The following are some of the crucial factors to take into account when choosing an HIS:**
> - **Total cost of the package:** In general, HIS providers are pleased to come and talk to you about the needs of your hospital. Hospitals of diverse sizes and financial capacities can find solutions. A hospital information system that has a low total cost of ownership is crucial. By creating a design that uses less hardware, some vendors can lower costs. This kind of design is known to lower long-term maintenance expenses while simultaneously lowering up-front acquisition costs.
> - **Web-based system:** A good HIS system needs to be accessible online in addition to having user-friendly features. Because the information is available online, authorized personnel can access it from any location and at any time. This frees up caregivers from being confined to office workstations and gives them information when they most need it. If information is shared across two or more hospitals, a web-based system becomes even more crucial. If healthcare facilities adopt an internet-based HIS, they can instantly transmit pertinent data across different geographic areas. For better care or specialized treatment, a hospital could elect to transfer a patient to another facility.
> - **Implementation and support:** Humans are always resistant to change, and implementing or upgrading a medical information system could result in backlash from staff members. It is always preferable to request staff training as well as implementation support from the vendor. Select a vendor that provides telephone or online support available around-the-clock so your hospital staff can get help right away. Some hospitals will also speak with their employees before making a purchase decision, because they could be able to share new information with you or alert you to details that others might have missed.
> - **User-friendly:** The user interface needs to be clear and simple.

Examples of Healthcare Information Systems

Electronic Medical Record (EMR) and Electronic Health Records (EHR)

The clinic's computer systems store a patient's permanent electronic medical record (EMR). This file, which is mostly utilized by primary care physicians and specialists, may include information about a patient's family history, allergies, medications, diagnoses, surgery information, and progress notes. Even though EHR can be thought of as a digital record that performs all that EMR does and more, these records might still need to be printed out in order to be shared with other medical professionals.

Several doctors and healthcare organizations outside of a practize utilise EHR to organize patient data.

Systems for Clinical Information (CIS)

Rapid information collection, archiving, processing, and distribution to decision-makers are the main objectives of clinical information systems (CIS). CIS is mostly utilized by hospitals and can include health histories, medications, doctor's notes, dictation, and any other information that is preserved together electronically (labs, pharmacies, radiology, and ICU). The main benefit of this system is its capacity to interface with other systems and exchange data with other instruments.

Practice Management Software (PMS)

Many allied healthcare professionals utilize practise management software, including psychologists, physiotherapists, and nurses. The use of a PMS makes it easier to manage a clinic's daily activities, such as online scheduling, billing, patient reminders, and other administrative tasks. Depending on the type of medical practise the software is developed for, practise management systems' features can change. Additional elements that are typically included with PMS include clinical notes, video sessions, online forms, links, and patient payments.

Patient Registries

A patient portal enables online access to the patient's personal information, including previous appointments, medical history, diagnoses, and more. Any internet-connected device, whether a mobile phone, desktop computer, laptop, or tablet, can normally access a patient portal around-the-clock. Patients can also set up appointments and have direct conversations with their medical personnel.

Master Patient Index (MPI)

The Master Patient Index (MPI) is an electronic database that assigns patients a special identifying number based on their geographic location, facilitating cross-referencing between healthcare systems and providers, including hospitals, doctors, labs, and imaging centers. Keeping patient data in the system allows for more effective and efficient transmission of medical records. For instance, a patient who is pregnant may need several healthcare services throughout their pregnancy and will need to see a range of healthcare specialists, including their doctor, OB, midwife, and laboratory technician.

Remote Patient Observation

Remote patient monitoring reduces hospital readmissions by allowing individuals to regularly use a medical gadget and evaluate their health outside of a clinic or hospital. In 2016, 7 million people employed this technology as part of their care; it is anticipated that 50 million people will do so in five years. These tools can keep an eye on things like:
- Unhealthy weight gain or loss
- High or low blood pressure
- Increasing or decreasing sugar levels
- Unusual oxygen saturation values

This makes it possible for healthcare professionals to remotely check on patients' health and status updates and use video conferencing to enhance patient care in general.

Tools for Clinical Decision Support

Clinical decision support (CDS) systems can notify healthcare professionals of information that they could be missing and foresee future issues, such as a patient who is dangerously combining medications. By recommending "next actions" based on a significant amount of digital data, they can assist clinicians in making judgments regarding treatments.

HOSPITAL INFORMATION SYSTEM

All information processing as well as the associated human or technology actors in their respective information processing roles make up the socio-technical subsystem of a hospital known as the hospital information system. For the purpose of managing patient care and related administrative chores, a hospital will implement a hospital information management system. The system's total efficiency may be improved by automation, which also generates the crucial project reports needed for controlling operations, performance, quality, planning, and reporting.

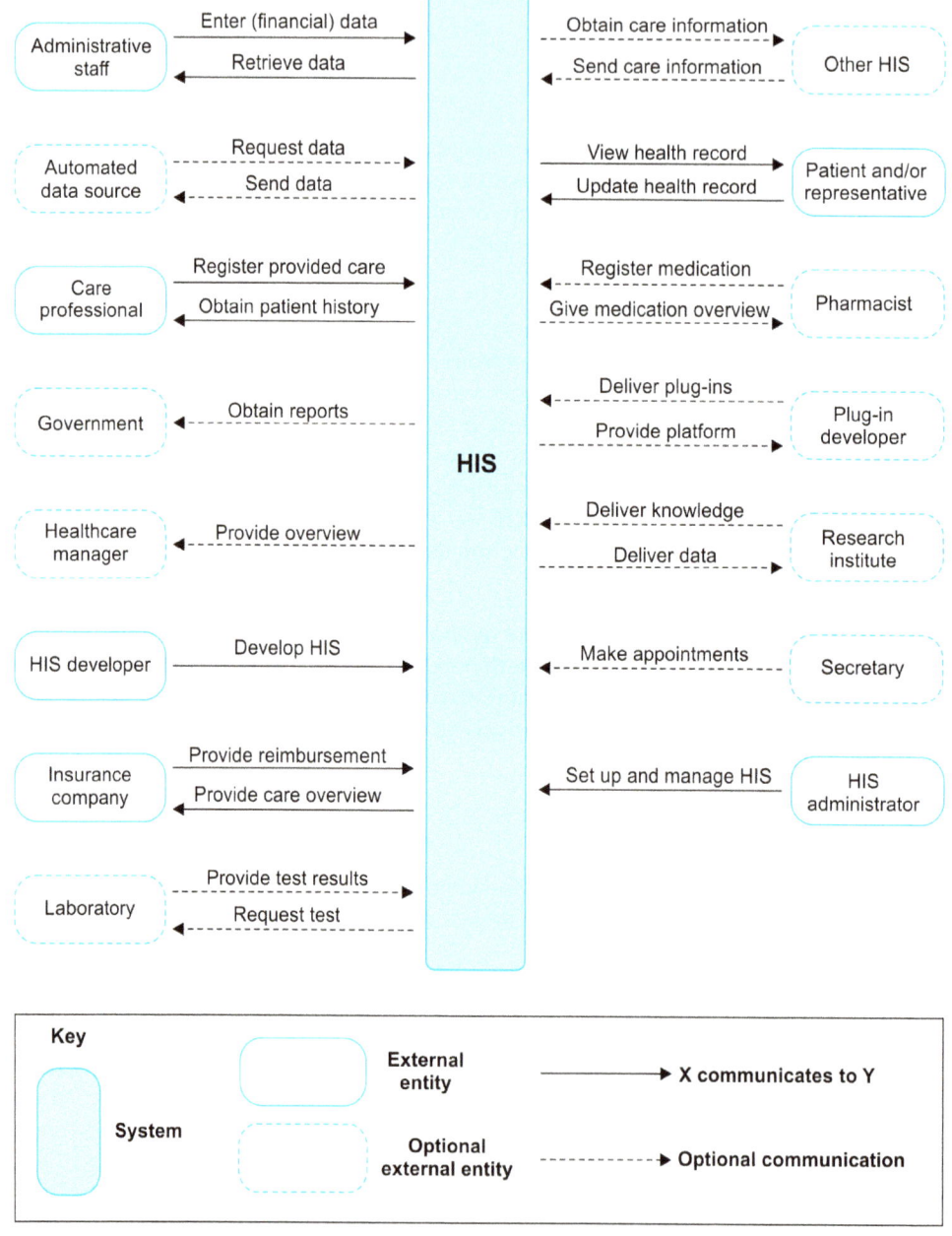

Fig. 3.6: HIS communication flow.

Information System in Healthcare

Hospital information systems (HIS), a subset of health informatics, are primarily focused on the administrative needs of hospitals. An HIS is frequently a comprehensive, integrated information system designed to manage all facets of a hospital's operations, including the processing of services in compliance with medical, administrative, financial, and legal considerations. Other names for the same thing include hospital management system (HMS) and hospital information system.

Healthcare providers, on the other hand, have recently altered their behaviour and are looking into all available angles that allow ICT to enhance managerial operations and the quality of healthcare while remaining affordable. This is because there is an unprecedented amount of competition and pressure to increase the effectiveness and quality of care. The HCISs, which are composed of numerous systems, should be integrated and coordinated as a whole, in accordance with this new point of view, to support treatment in an organizational and procedural framework that is patient-centric. HCISs are thus in a unique position to receive, store, process, and transmit timely information to decision-makers for better healthcare coordination at all of the aforementioned levels of analysis.

Definition

Any quantitative and qualitative data that might help doctors and health decision-makers better understand disease processes and healthcare difficulties, as well as to prevent, identify, and treat health issues, is considered to be health information. An information system for managing a health programme or system and keeping track of health-related activities consists of interconnected component elements for collecting, processing, and distributing information (management information, health statistics, and health literature).

It is the information system that gathers, stores, processes, retrieves, and communicates patient care and administrative information using computers, communication tools, and software.

AIMS OF HOSPITAL INFORMATION SYSTEM

- To ensure that electronic data processing provides the best possible assistance for patient care and administration.
- In order to give patients the best care, results, and administration, networked electronic data processing is used to capture data as it is generated and show it where it is needed.
- Accurate data storage, reliable usage, quick access to data, secure data storage, and reduced usage costs are the main objectives for hospital information systems.
- Information regarding a patient's medical history is centralized in hospital information systems.
- These systems help healthcare practitioners better organize patient care.
- HIS help healthcare providers communicate both internally and outside. The HIS may be used to manage organizations, in this case a hospital, and their official paperwork, financial situation reports, personal information, utility bills, and stock levels. It also maintains secure patient records for medical histories, prescriptions, operations, and laboratory test results.
- The HIS may defend organizations from faults in official documents, such as mistakes in tax preparation, overstock issues, and scheduling conflicts.

History of hospital information system	Events
1970s	Began mostly with financial systems, offering assistance to the company's billing, payroll, accounting, and reporting systems Radiology, laboratory and pharmacy
1980s	With significant expenditures in systems for cost accounting and materials management, financial systems rose to prominence once more
1990s	Healthcare systems that are used throughout an organization, such as clinical data archives and ideas for a completely computerized electronic medical record (EMR)

Benefits of HIS

- Efficient and precise management of finances, patient food, engineering, and medical aid distribution.
- Having a broad perspective on hospital expansion is beneficial.
- Better drug monitoring and efficacy research that reduces unfavorable drug interactions while encouraging more sensible use of pharmaceuticals.
- Hospital software is simple to use and eliminates errors brought on by handwriting. It also improves information integrity, lowers transcribing errors, and minimizes duplication of information entries. Computers using cutting-edge technology function flawlessly while retrieving data from servers or cloud servers.
- A quicker and better reaction from the healthcare system, instant connection to experts and other service providers.
- Using computerized clinical applications, healthcare is more affordable.
- In an emergency anywhere in the globe, data is instantaneously available thanks to electronic medical records.
- Reduces extra time and travel for medical professionals, and aids in automatically monitoring for drug and other interactions.

WHO BENEFITS FROM HOSPITAL INFORMATION SYSTEM?

The staff and patients, computer users, and administrative staff can all provide information on the hospital information system. Hospital information systems can be identified by their advantages, functions, types of processed data, and types of services they provide. The groups listed below gain from hospital information systems:

Physicians

- Expands the use of computerized provider order entry (CPOE)
- Enhances the access to and accuracy of the necessary patient drugs
- Enhances care through the logging of all orders
- Reduces medication error rates
- Enhances clinicians' efficiency and effectiveness by providing crucial patient information (such as allergies) at the time of ordering, as well as conflict checking, order checking, and online access to best practise information

Nurses and Allied Health Professionals

- Gives quick access to orders and outcomes
- Gives quick access to patient details, prescription information, and test results
- Enables easier online information access (i.e., suggested medications or drug alerts)
- Reduce the use of paper, cut down on errors, and improve patient safety
- Reduces the need for paper, reduces mistakes, and improves patient safety

Ward and Registration Clerks

Reduces duplication of work by providing a single point of contact for patient registration information.

Clinical Benefits

- When and where they are needed, healthcare personnel will be able to access a patient's health information and visit history, which will improve their ability to coordinate care.
- The EPR will be integrated with information from diagnostic information systems like X-ray and laboratory, improving internal and external communication among healthcare practitioners. The EPR will eventually be applicable everywhere.
- Permit medical staff to access a patient's medical records from different facilities.

Administrative Benefits

- Reduces the need for paper, cuts down on mistakes, and makes it easier to find information online, (e.g., suggested prescriptions or drug alerts).
- Lessen the need for patients to re-register at various sites through improving internal and external communication among healthcare professionals.

SUBSYSTEMS OF HIS

The usage of hospital information systems is part of a "integrated effort to gather, process, report, and apply health information and knowledge to impact policy-making, programme action, and research." HISs come in a variety of forms, including routine- and clinical-HISs. A hospital information system's components include two or more of the following:

Picture Archiving and Communication System (PACS)

A PACS is a type of medical imaging system that enables the affordable storage and simple transfer of images from many modalities (source machine types). PACS does away with the need to physically file, retrieve, or move film jackets by transferring digitized images and reports digitally. PACS images can only be stored and transferred in the DICOM format (Digital Imaging and Communications in Medicine). Non-image data, such as scanned documents, may be added using consumer industry standard formats like PDF after being contained in DICOM (Portable Document Format). A PACS is made up of four key components: imaging methods including computed tomography, magnetic resonance, and plain-film X-rays.

Information System in Healthcare

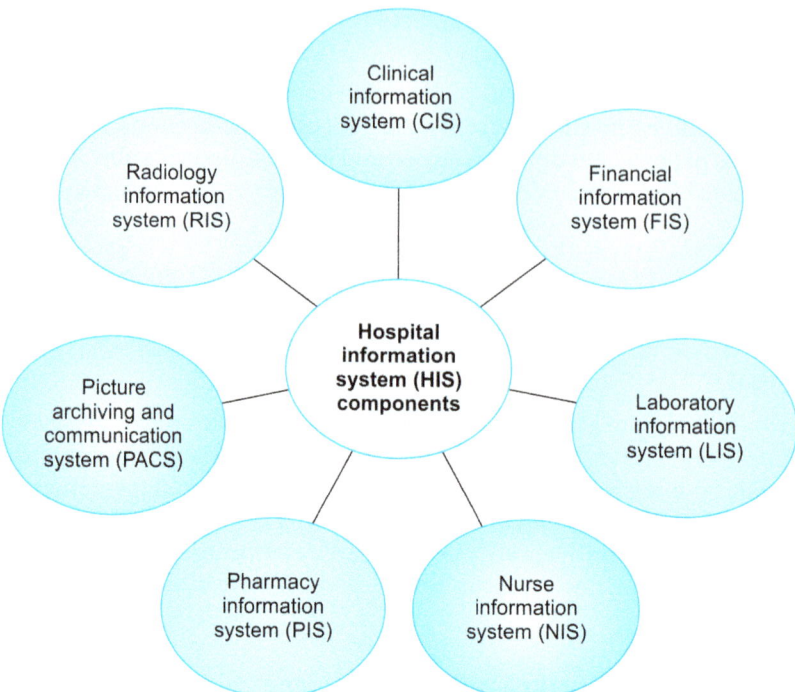

Fig. 3.7: HIS components.

Imaging, as well as a secure network for transmitting patient data, workstations for analyzing and evaluating images, and archives for the storage and retrieval of images and reports.

Radiology Information System (RIS)

These systems' capacity to offer radiological billing services, appointment scheduling, reporting, and patient information storage makes them popular as well. Technology advancements have made radiology practises more complex, and many institutions are increasingly using RIS to run the business side of their businesses.

Clinical Information Systems (CIS)

A clinical information system is a computer-based platform created for the collection, storage, manipulation, and dissemination of clinical data vital to the delivery of healthcare. Healthcare organizations can enhance the provision of clinical services with the aid of clinical information systems. Clinical data and reports are presented through hospital information systems, allowing doctors to make more informed choices at the point of care. An information system called a clinical information system (CIS) is made expressly for use in critical care settings like intensive care units (ICU). It may connect to the several computer systems in a contemporary hospital, including radiology and pathology. It compiles data from every one of these programmes into an electronic patient record that doctors can access at the patient's bedside.

Benefits of a Clinical Information System

A CIS can help patients and clinicians by:
- Enhancing communication among the numerous healthcare providers who provide care for each patient;
- Giving clinicians all the data they need to make wise decisions;
- Simplifying the process for patients to have X-rays and scans when necessary;
- Encouraging quality improvement; and
- Facilitating better clinical research.

Clinical Information Systems in Intensive Care

ICUs use a variety of medical instruments to continuously monitor seriously ill patients. There is a huge volume of information production. Clinicians can make the best choices with the help of this knowledge. As opposed to roughly 32 clinical measurements per day per patient in a standard ward, it is estimated that ICU clinicians manage about 1700 clinical measurements each day per patient.

The majority of these metrics must be taken by doctors without a CIS, who then document them on paper-based, 24-hour "ICU flow charts."

All of these measurements can be electronically recorded, collected, and captured using a CIS. This decreases the need for numerous paper forms, saves time, and lowers the possibility of error.

Nursing Information Systems (NIS)

To assist nurses in giving patients better care, these computer-based information systems were created. A strong NIS may carry out a variety of tasks and provide advantages like better staff schedules, accurate patient charting, and improved clinical data integration. Through schedule apps that allow managers to handle absences and overtime, the nursing department's workforce can be more effectively managed. A more cost-effective staffing strategy can be achieved by using the solution to monitor personnel levels. Applications for patient charting let users enter information about patients' vital signs. It is also used by nurses for admission details, treatment plans, and any pertinent nursing notes. All significant information is safely kept and is accessible when needed. Clinical data integration is also incredibly helpful, since it enables nurses to gather, access, and analyse clinical data before integrating it to create a patient's care plan. In the end, all of these NIS aspects result in shorter planning times and more accurate assessments and evaluations. Since, there is always a reference for pharmaceuticals that are prescribed electronically, the likelihood of prescribing the incorrect treatment diminishes as well.

Physician Information Systems (PIS)

PIS systems, as their name suggests, are suggested for use by the government and aim to enhance medical practitioners' practises. The federal government's stimulus package, which aims to improve healthcare, is available to doctors. Different packages are available to fit different budgets and can be used to boost productivity, reduce expenses, and provide high-quality patient care. Electronic medical records (EMRs), electronic health records (EHRs), and other commonly used and well-liked apps are used by physician information systems, which are given through computers, servers, and networks. The majority of these programmes offer round-the-clock remote help, enabling hospital staff to diagnose issues that arise while using the system.

Pharmacy Information Systems (PIS)

PIS assists pharmacists in keeping track of the way medication is used in hospitals and was created to meet the expectations of a pharmacy department. PIS aids consumers in managing drug allergies and other side effects of medications. The method helps give the right medications depending on the patient's physiologic variables and enables users to identify drug interactions.

Financial Information System (FIS)

Computer programmes called financial information systems are used to run a hospital's financial operations. Even though healthcare organizations' top priority is saving lives rather than generating profits, they do incur running costs from daily operations, such as purchases and employee salaries.

Laboratory Information System (LIS)

A software-based laboratory and information management system known as a laboratory information management system (LIMS), also known as a laboratory information system (LIS) or laboratory management system (LMS), provides a number of essential features that support the operations of a modern laboratory.

INFORMATION SYSTEM FOR PATIENT CARE

The hospital information system (HIS) can be broadly divided into two halves:
1. Systems for the patient care function
2. Managerial information systems

A group of systems that can be collectively referred to as information systems for the patient care function support the clinical and other patient care-related functions. Although the phrase "patient care information system" is appealing and appropriate, it is regrettably only utilized by a tiny number of supporters. Since using this extra category level as the parent and the clinical information system (CIS) as the child clarifies the nomenclature, it will be used in all upcoming conversations. Not all information systems for patient care are referred to as clinical information systems. Instead, the system that supports or promotes direct patient care functions alone bears the name CIS. The other half of the system is the information systems for clinical support services which are made up of several modules.

Patient Care Information System

EMR/EHR systems is a phrase that is frequently used. Since information systems are only helpful if they make work easier rather than just "the development, storage, and management of electronic medical data," as some people understand it, this term is misleading and shouldn't be used at all.

Patient Care Information System—Objectives and Functions

These subsystems and applications, which serve as a system for streamlining operations, are anticipated to make best use of computerization and information technology to achieve the following goals:
- Productivity
- Effectiveness
- Appropriateness
- Efficiency

Information System in Healthcare

- Quality
- Safety
- Privacy and confidentiality of information

To achieve the above objectives, the computerized information system is required to provide the following functions:
- Facilitate and direct the execution of patient care processes.
- Enable automation of work processes by connecting to other computers, devices, printers, and scanners as well as other components of the hospital information system.
- Promote communication between healthcare providers through information exchange.
- Offer point-of-care clinical decision support.
- For use in primary and secondary applications, compile, preserve, and make available essential clinical data (both individual and aggregated).
- Keep an archive of all events and patient care activities (as the electronic medical record and other documents based on medico-legal requirements)
- Any system that is being developed, advocated, or implemented must possess characteristics that would satisfy all of the aforementioned goals and functions, both in terms of the information it contains and the methods it employs.

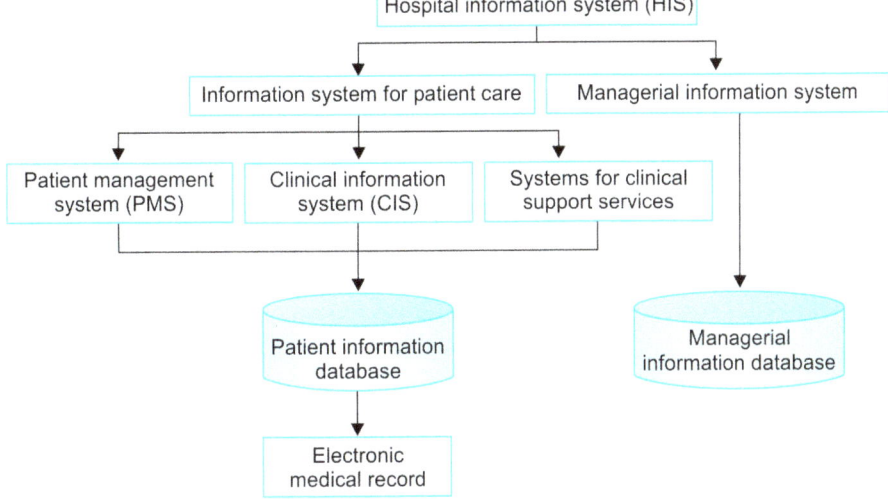

Fig. 3.8: Classification of hospital information system.

CLINICAL INFORMATION SYSTEM

The clinical information system (CIS) supports activities where healthcare professionals, primarily physicians and nurses, but also dietitians, therapists, clinical psychologists, clinical pharmacists, clinical microbiologists, interventional radiologists, endoscopists, optometrists, and audiologist, among many others, directly care for patients. Along with gathering relevant data generated, a competent CIS aids and directs physicians in carrying out their duties.

The CIS includes application modules (whatever their names may be) that permit:
- Care planning (use of care plans)
- Availability of clinical decision aid
- Clinical data recording (data entry)
- Quality assurance
- Storage of data

Information System in Healthcare

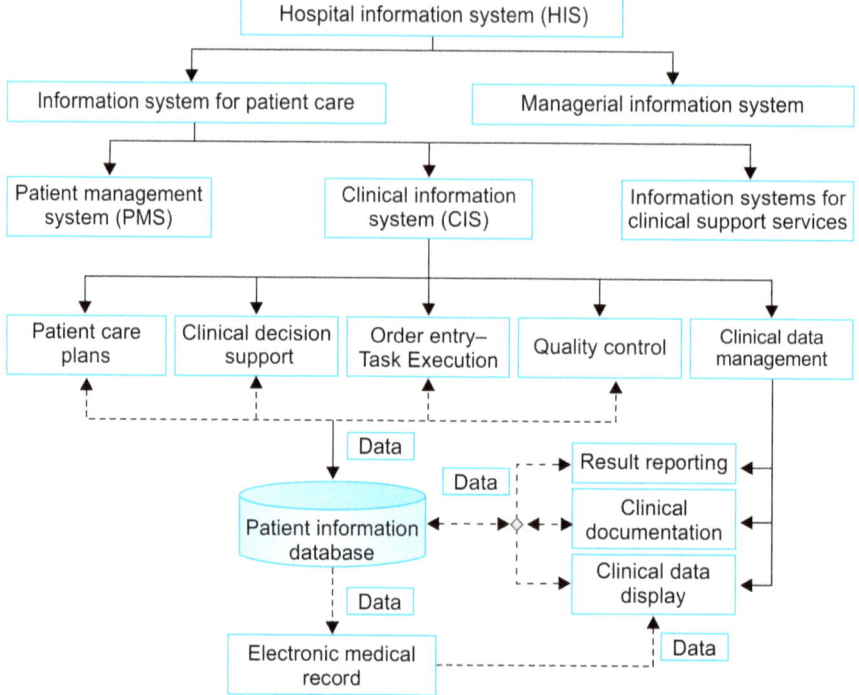

Fig. 3.9: Components of the clinical information system.

SYSTEMS FOR CLINICAL SUPPORT

Services that perform tests and offer supplies are referred to as clinical support.

Through the order entry feature, direct care providers request these services. The database receives test results, which are then made accessible from there. Drugs, blood products, sterile supplies, and meals are supplied to individuals or units that have requested them. The database contains information about their delivery and receipt.

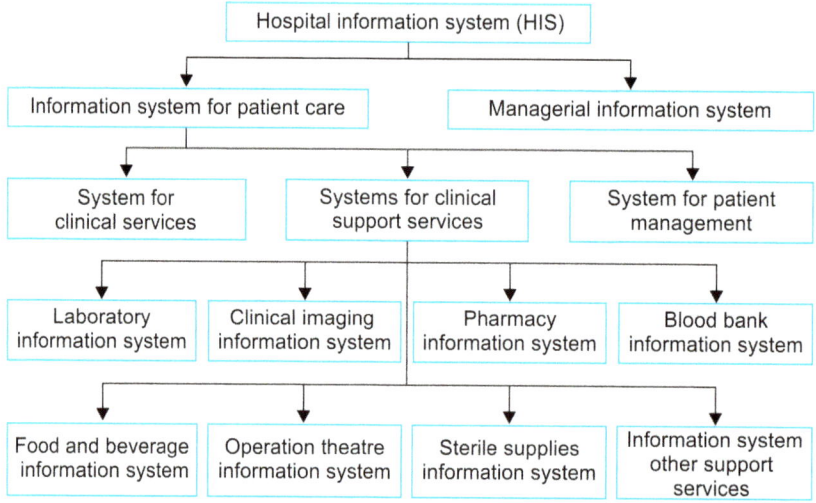

Fig. 3.10: System for clinical support services.

INTEGRATION OF THE COMPONENTS PATIENT CARE INFORMATION SYSTEM

Integration is crucial within the Patient Care Information System. The right links between this system's subsystems and modules are essential to its efficient operation. When purchasing, it is ideal if they are already completely integrated.

Key Applications for Bridging

The Clinical Information System and the different Clinical Support Systems, which are the primary patient care applications software, are constructed around important bridge (intermediary) components such as:

❏ Patient administration/management system (registration, scheduling, resource allocation)
❏ Order-entry result reporting application (CPOE)
❏ Database management system (DBMS)
❏ Electronic medical record
❏ A common user-system interface

These applications are first considered and created, and as each clinical and clinical-support application is created, they are modified. These essential bridge (intermediary) apps are interoperable with other software programmes.

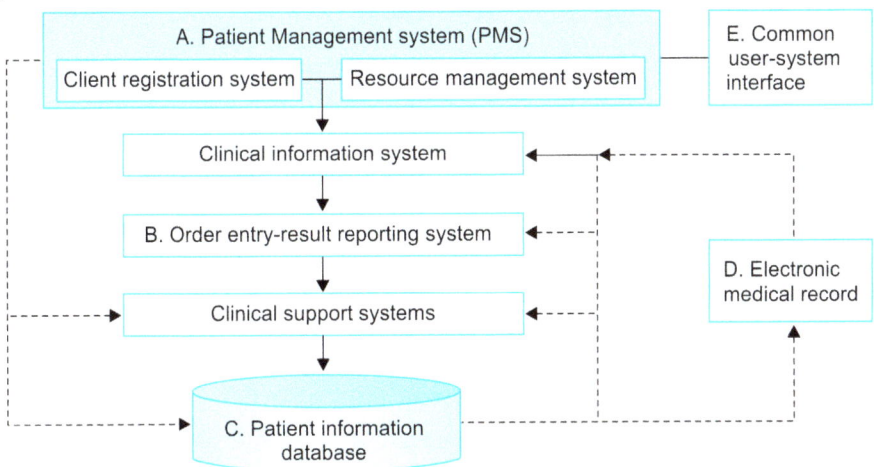

Fig. 3.11: Bridging of the patient care information system.

ROLE OF PATIENT ADMINISTRATION/MANAGEMENT SYSTEM (PMS)

The patient information database receives identity, demographic, and other static data from the patient administration/management system (PMS), such as payment class. These data are derived by other systems from the database, assuring their standardization and eliminating the need for recurrent acquisition.

Information System in Healthcare

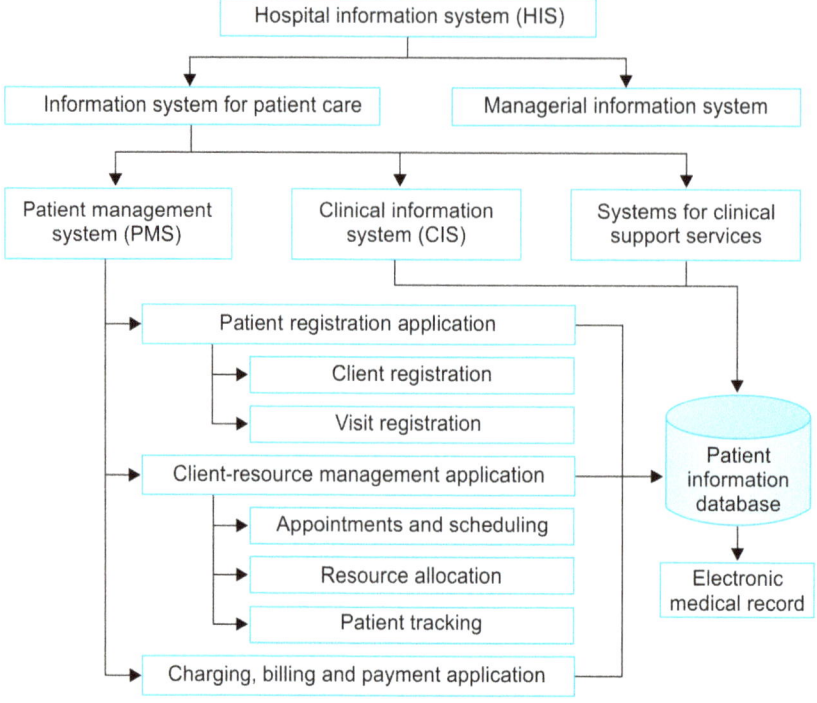

Fig. 3.12: Role of HIS.

COMPONENTS OF MANAGERIAL INFORMATION SYSTEM

Systems that support the business operations include:
- General administration information system and office automation
- Charging, billing and receipt of payment (accounting) system
- Human resources management system
- Finance and budgetary systems
- Consumables purchasing and inventory system

Systems for facilitating the hospitality services of a hospital include:
- Bed management
- Food-beverage order-supply system

Systems for management of the hospital as a physical facility include:
- Facility engineering systems
- Equipment and machinery maintenance and inventory system
- Environmental safety, housekeeping, cleansing and waste management

Managerial decision support systems (DSS) can be very helpful and include:
- Business management decision support
- Clinical governance decision support

The DSS may have a range of capabilities. Simple statistical tools to business intelligence software are all possible. Large firms can also want to use enterprise resource planning software and build a data warehouse.

Information System in Healthcare

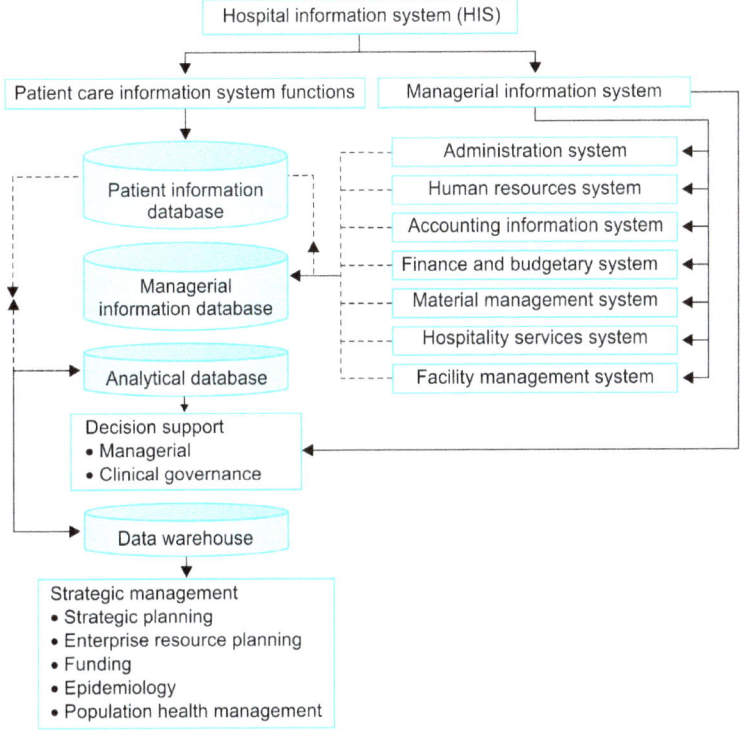

Fig. 3.13: Managerial information system.

The managerial information system is made up of numerous, intricate components. Although they are not currently the focus of this conversation, they are included here for completeness. But we'll talk about some of the parts that interface or integrate with the information system for patient care function.

Hospital Information System Portal

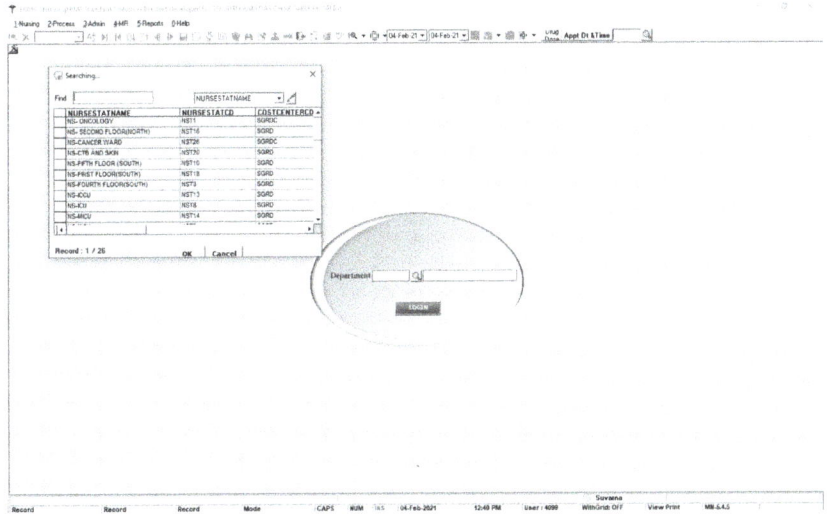

Information System in Healthcare

Login and Searching in the System

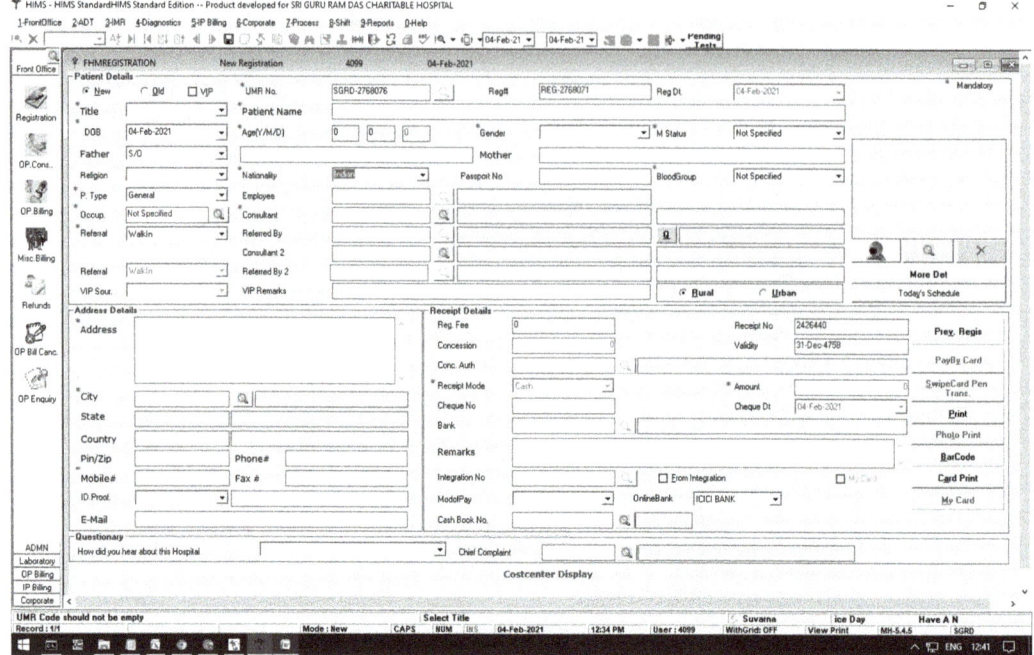

Electronic Medical Record

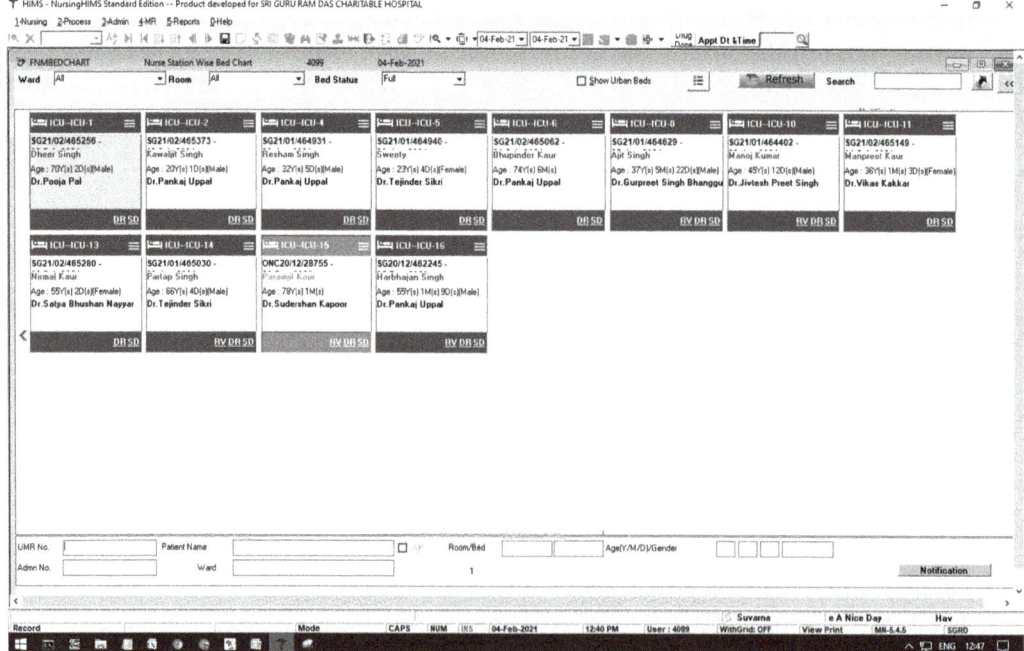

Information System in Healthcare

Patient Bed Chart (Patient Bedwise Services)

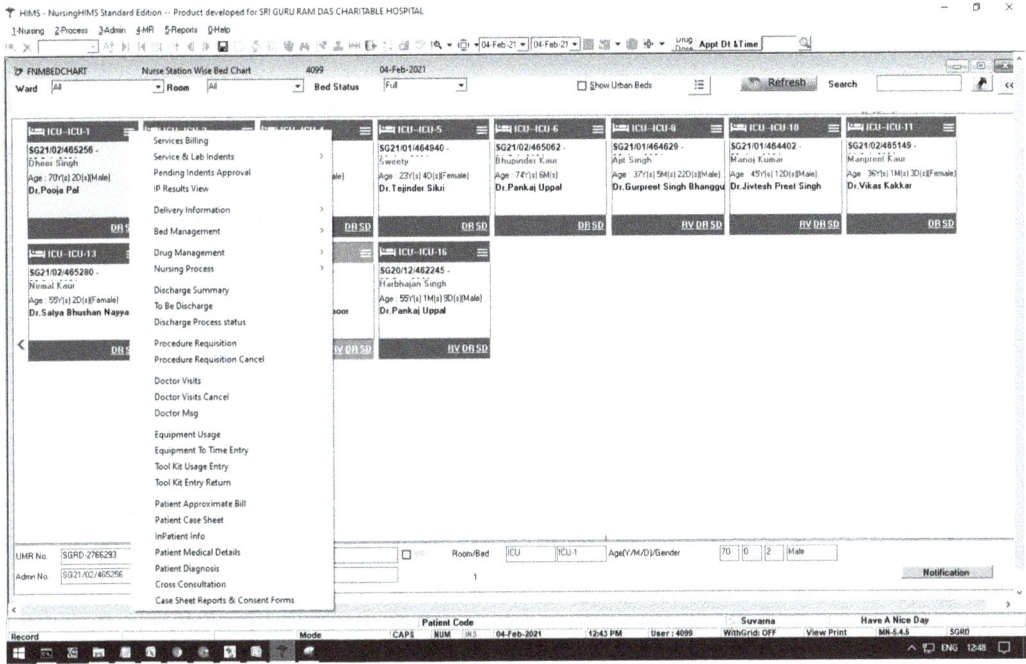

Patient Bedwise Notification

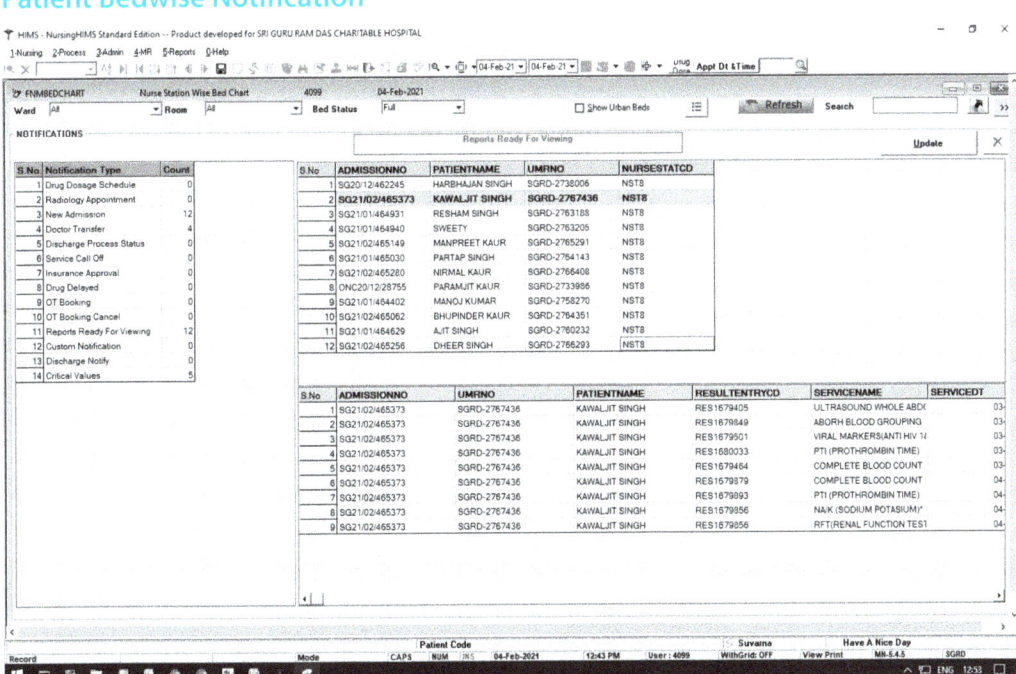

Patient Consultation

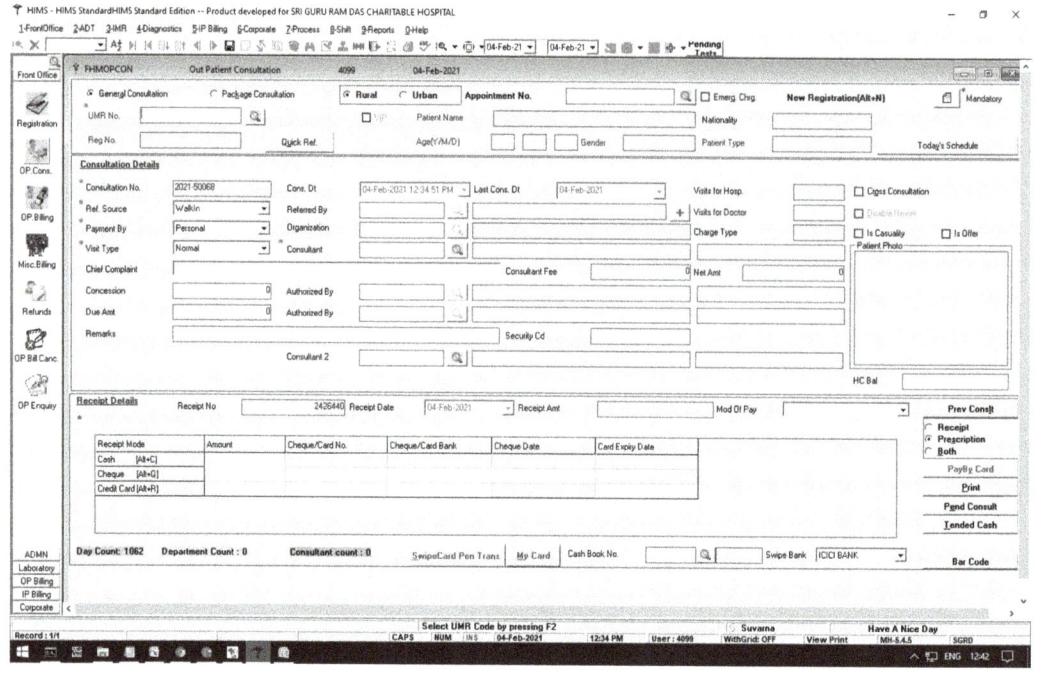

Patient Billing

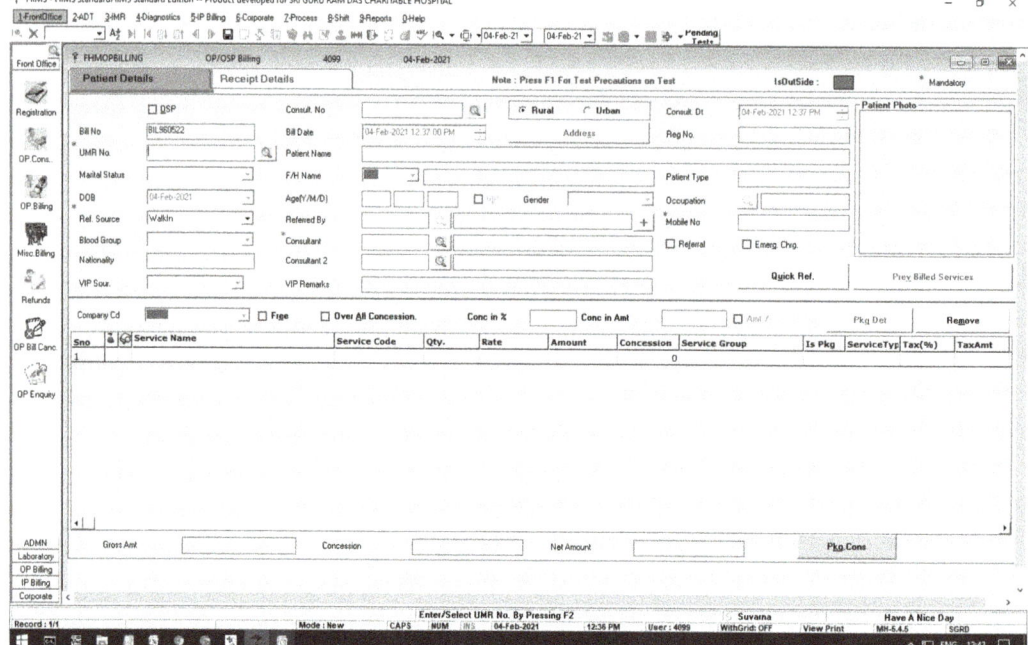

Information System in Healthcare

Patient OPD Slip

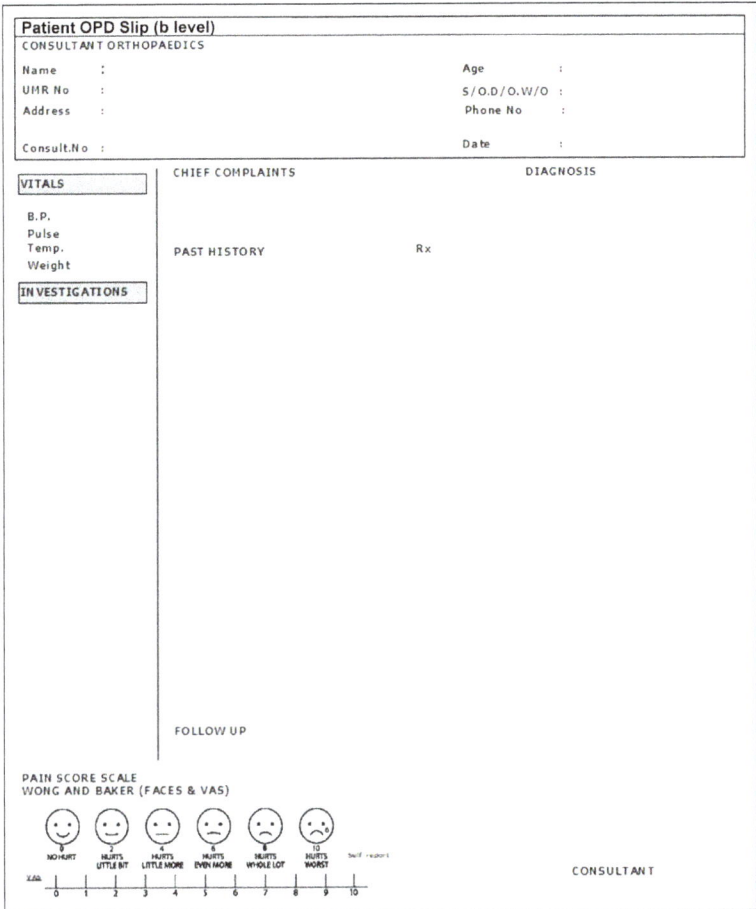

Patient Investigation Billing Record

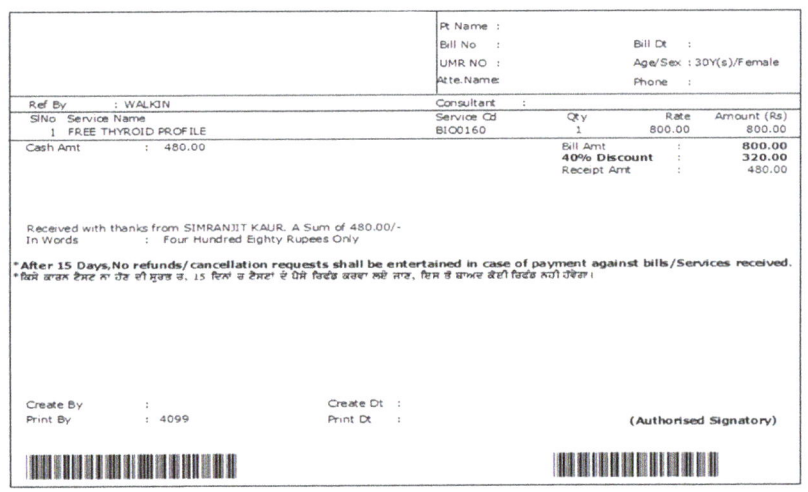

SUMMARY

A system created to manage healthcare data is referred to as a "health information system" (HIS). This comprises the operational administration of a hospital or a system that supports the formulation of healthcare policy, as well as systems that gather, store, manage, and transmit a patient's electronic medical record (EMR).

Systems that manage data relevant to the operations of providers and healthcare organizations are also included in the category of health information systems. These could be used in concert to impact research, enhance patient outcomes, and improve policy and decision-making. Security is a top priority since health information systems frequently access, handle, or keep significant volumes of sensitive data.

REVIEW QUESTION

1. Describe the architecture of HIS.
2. Discuss briefly roles of information system in healthcare.
3. Enlist the components of typical HIS architecture.
4. What are the components of HIS? Discuss briefly.
5. Write the points needed while selecting a effective HIS.
6. What are the aims of hospital information system?
7. Elaborate the benefits of HIS.
8. Discuss the examples of healthcare information system.
9. Discuss about patient care information in details.
10. What is clinical information system and its uses?

MULTIPLE CHOICE QUESTIONS

1. **What is a comprehensive technology system that allows hospitals to manage all aspects of operation?**
   a. Health information system
   b. Hospital information system
   c. Managerial information system
   d. Hospital management model

2. **What type of management system include patient scheduling?**
   a. Core system
   b. Business system
   c. Finance system
   d. Medical systems

3. **Without healthcare data and information, their would be no need for healthcare information.**
   a. True
   b. False

4. **Healthcare organizations maintain medical record for one primary purpose.**
   a. True
   b. False

5. **Which of the following is not a component of HIS?**
   a. Patient archieving system
   b. Pharmacy information system
   c. Nursing information system
   d. Community information system

6. **Which of the following department carries out the filing, retrieving and indexing of records?**
   a. Maintenance department
   b. Therapeutic
   c. Medical records department
   d. Administration department

7. **The backbone of the hospital organization and the hospital information system is:**
   a. Financial and economic resources
   b. Planned architecture of hospital information system
   c. Components of HIS
   d. Stakeholders

8. **The objectives of management information system is all, *except*:**
   a. Support clinical decision-making
   b. Recruitment of manpower
   c. Provide information required at each level
   d. Facilitate decision-making

9. **The logical design of information system is translated into physical structure which includes hardware, software, network support and processing methods is called…**
   a. Database server
   b. Analytical domain
   c. Web network
   d. System architecture

10. **Which of the following is essential while selecting HIS architecture?**
    a. Web based system
    b. Data frame
    c. Corporate portals
    d. Legacy system

11. **Which of the following design locates all or most of the processing logic on the server?**
    a. Topological client
    b. Portal client
    c. Thick client
    d. Thin client

Answer Key

1. b
2. d
3. a
4. b
5. d
6. c
7. b
8. b
9. d
10. a
11. d

CHAPTER 4

Shared Care and Electronic Health Records

At the end of this chapter, student will able to learn about:
- Electronic health records
- Features of electronics health records
- Challenges related to electronic health records implementation.
- How to implement successful electronic health record system
- Goals of electronic health records standards
- Latest trends in electronic health records
- Benefits of electronic medical records
- Standard for electronic health records

TERMINOLOGIES

- **Protected health information (PHI):** Protected Health Information (PHI) is any data about a person's health status, the delivery of healthcare, or payment for healthcare that was generated or gathered by a covered entity.
- **Electronic health record (EHR):** An electronic version of a patient's medical history that is kept up to date over time by the healthcare provider. It may include all of the essential administrative clinical data relevant to that person's care under a specific provider, such as demographics, progress notes, issues, medications, vital signs, past medical histories, immunizations, laboratory information, and radiology reports.
- **Electronic medical record (EMR):** An antiquated but still used word. It now generally refers to the software's actual clinical features, including those that screen for drug interactions, allergies, encounter documentation, etc.

INTRODUCTION

The healthcare industry has seen an increase in worldwide technical innovation in recent decades. The electronic health record is one excellent illustration of this. The fast evolution of the electronic health record over a little period of time has made it an indispensable platform for using and sharing health information. In order to improve patient outcomes through safety and quality of care, it is utilized all over the world as a means of sharing health information across different healthcare professionals, tracking a patient's progress, and trending test findings. One of the most significant technological developments, the electronic health record serves as a quicker and more secure replacement for the conventional handwritten paper charts.

The complexity that comes with using technological platforms, however, means that experts have to spend more time dealing with it. The time it takes to operate devices and technology, time that could have been spent providing direct and indirect patient care through nursing chores at the bedside, is a problem that healthcare personnel frequently run into. Although the World Health Organization acknowledges the value of electronic health records, more study is still required to guarantee that moral, secure, and high quality criteria are upheld.

ELECTRONIC HEALTH RECORDS

Electronic health records refer to storing patient data and information on a digital platform, such as a computer, so that authorized hospital employees can access and use it. It covers the patient's diagnosis, course of treatment, drugs, lab results, and any other pertinent data.

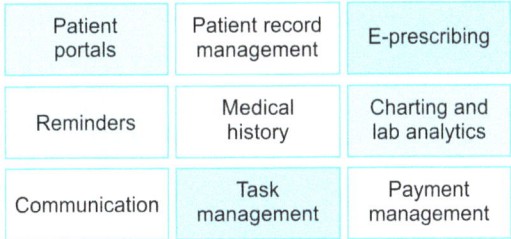

Fig. 4.1: Features of electronic health records.

Patient Portals

A patient portal contains information of patient, such as:

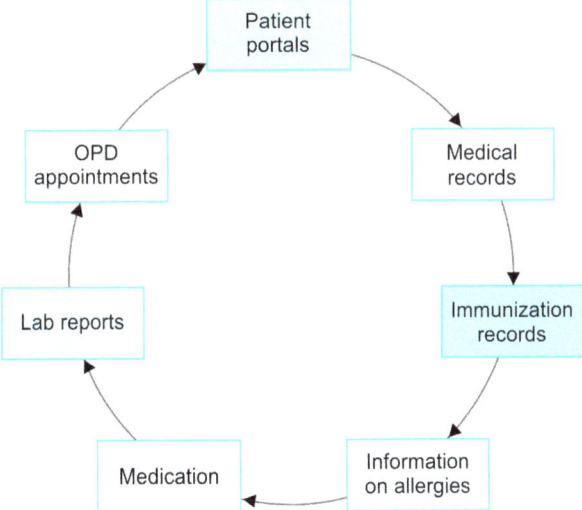

Fig. 4.2: Patient information system on e-records.

Patient Record Management

Patient record management consists of **Figure 4.3**.

E-Prescribing

Software for electronic health records may offer an e-prescribing capability that allows a doctor to electronically give a patient's prescription.

In place of paper prescriptions and faxed prescriptions, electronic prescribing is the computer-based generation, transmission, and filling of a medical prescription. A doctor or nurse practitioner can electronically transmit a fresh prescription by using e-prescribing.

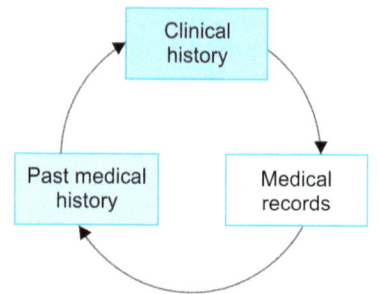

Fig. 4.3: Patient record management system.

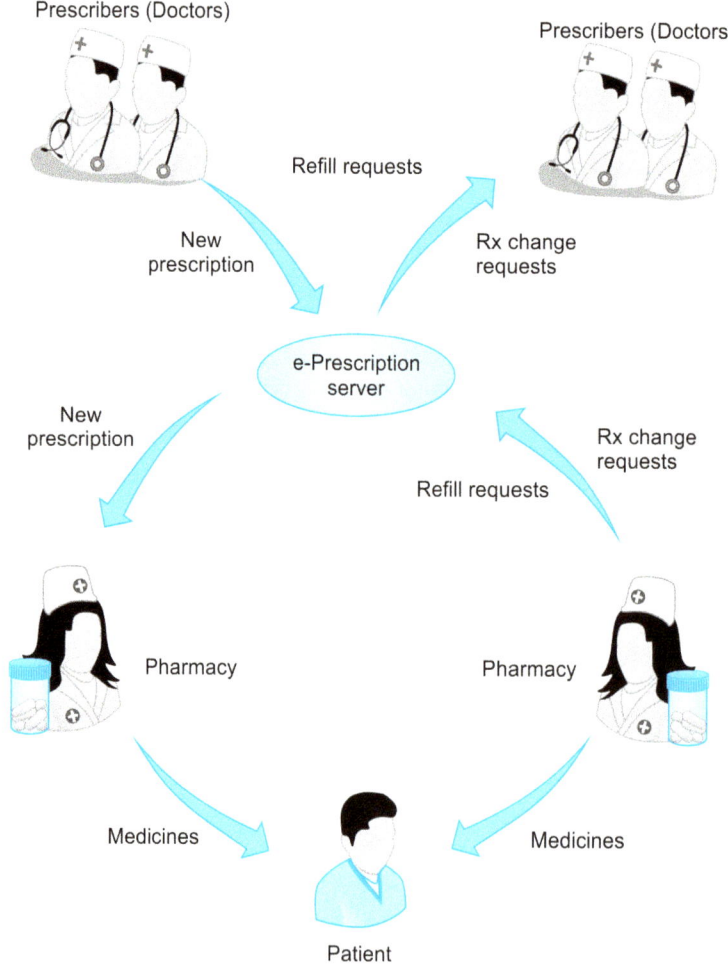

Fig. 4.4: E-Prescription process.

Medical History

The medical history feature in an EHR will include:
- Past medical conditions
- Specific medical problems
- Treatments given in the past

CHALLENGES RELATED TO ELECTRONIC HEALTH RECORDS IMPLEMENTATION

- **Implementation cost:** The cost of electronic health records in healthcare settings is somewhat high. Not all hospitals have the financial means to set up, implement, and optimize electronic patient records. Everything is dependent on the healthcare organization's finances. Unexpected costs may also arise during the implementation. One of the biggest obstacles to EHR deployment is finding the necessary funding, especially for smaller companies. Implementation of electronic health records needs following planning:
  - Setting up the hardware
  - Software costs
  - Implementation assistance
  - Training for the staff
  - Ongoing network fees
  - Maintenance of data server
- **Staff reticence:** Not all medical staff members are on board with using such a database to store patient information. The effectiveness of such computerized records is in question. Few lack knowledge and require training to manage electronic records. The deployment of electronic health records is delayed as a result of all these factors. They might appear hesitant to abandon the documentation process. In certain circumstances, the workforce is unaware of the most recent technology developments and their many advantages.
- **Training takes time:** Because medical staff need specialized training to handle such things, implementing the electronic health records system is quite challenging. Programs for faculty growth or training take a lot of time, and extra time is required for system training. Small hospitals with little resources cannot afford to spend so much extra on systems and training.
- **Poor usability:** The adoption of electronic health records varies throughout departments since the workflows of a dentist and a cardiologist are different. This reduces the software's usability and makes it a little harder to adapt the system. The programme is less simple to use because of design defects or inadequate training.
- **Data privacy:** Data privacy and data leaks are another difficulty in the adoption of an electronic health record. Despite the fact that the stockholders express concern over the data breach caused by a cyber-attack. In case of a security breach, the healthcare business may get into legal issues. As a result, the provider now has a major duty to guarantee the electronic health records' data protection.
- **Data migration:** After electronic health records are implemented, the difficulty is to export the data from paper-based platforms to digital ones. Large amounts of paperwork detailing the medical histories of hundreds of patients will be present, making data entry a laborious and time-consuming operation for the hospital staff.
- **Technical resource limitations:** A hospital with a high budget can hire a technical team to manage the electronic record database, but small hospitals find it challenging to justify the cost of doing so. Building an internal technical staff and purchasing hardware is expensive,

which is a common justification given by small and mid-sized healthcare organizations for postponing the implementation of electronic record data.
- **Ineffective interoperability:** This is the inability of various electronic health record systems or software to exchange information so that various providers can use it. Inter-departmental networking is essential in electronic health record systems to obtain a complete picture of the client's health. Building an effective networking system that permits the movement of information among various providers is still a big challenge for healthcare providers. Not to add that appropriate care coordination between various providers is necessary for the client to have better health results.
- **Inadequate planning:** The introduction of electronic health records entails more of a culture shift within the company than a purely technical one. As a result, the introduction of electronic health records presents a significant barrier in terms of change management. All partners must be committed, and significant planning is required in preparation. Without extensive preparation, the successful implementation and sustainability of the electronic health records system would remain a pipe dream.
- **Poor communication:** Building an electronic health record system that produces excellent results requires two-way communication between the technical team and the healthcare provider. For the duration of the time period, it should be consistent to ensure that the technical requirements and expectations of healthcare personnel are met.

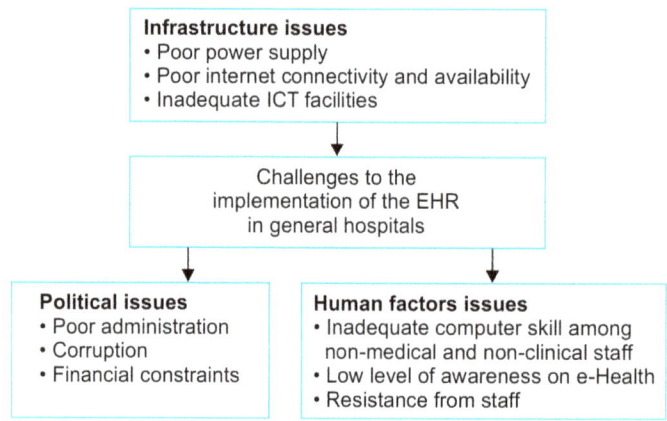

Fig. 4.5: Challenges related to electronic health records.

HOW TO IMPLEMENT SUCCESSFUL ELECTRONIC HEALTH RECORD SYSTEM?

- **Have a strategic strategy:** Creating a thorough strategic plan is the first step in implementing an electronic health record. Establish a team around the doctor who excels in technical tasks by assigning tasks and responsibilities to the team members. For individuals who are new to electronic health records, offer regular training and other incentives to pique their interest. Make sure the team has contingency plans in place and is prepared. During the implementation phase, staff productivity may drop, workflow may become chaotic, or even patients may become irritated. Here, it's crucial to keep in mind that successful adoption of electronic health records depends on planning.
- **Forms an interdisciplinary team:** The deployment of an electronic health record is a collaborative process that calls for the dedication of all team members, including software engineers, IT personnel, consultants, nurses, and medical professionals. Make the team's

collective goal to achieve the process larger vision a team goal. This facilitates timely, cost-effective, and usable implementation completion.
- **Ensure strong leadership:** Leaders should take aggressive measures to modify the management in order to build the team for the organization's implementation of electronic health records. To direct the implementation team, form a subcommittee of leaders with expertise in installing new IT systems in various disciplines.
- **Meet the deadline:** As the electronic health record implementation process is underway, meeting the deadlines can be difficult. By developing a practical plan, try to reduce timeline slippage as low as feasible. Inform your team of the cost to the implementation team of each day of delay.
- **Ensure adequate training:** The goal of using electronic health records is to increase effectiveness and efficiency. Make sure the personnel is properly trained. The objectives will remain unachievable if staff don't use the system properly and stick to the old ways of doing things. Utilize a thorough training programme for the employees, explain to them how the new system would improve patient care and make their jobs easier.

GOALS OF ELECTRONIC HEALTH RECORDS STANDARDS

The goals of electronic health records standard are as follows:
- Support the evolution and timely maintenance of records and e-portal.
- Promote technical innovation using adopted standards.
- Encourage participation and adoption by all vendors and stakeholders.
- Keep electronic health portal implementation cost as low as possible.
- Update the best practices and policies for electronic health records standards.

LATEST TRENDS IN ELECTRONIC RECORD TECHNOLOGY

The brain of a hospital is its medical records department, which is a developing division in the healthcare sector. The department maintains a database of all of the hospital's patients, both present and past. Medical professionals and hospitals can undoubtedly use well-kept medical records to their advantage when defending themselves in cases of malpractice. The majority of the time that healthcare workers are at work is spent on paperwork and standard operating procedures. When a patient enters a doctor's office, it's no longer necessary to dash down to a wet basement to dig through a stack of paper files.

Let us understand the recent advancements in this upcoming field:

Automated chatbots and voice messages: Automated chatbots and voice messages are available as standalone apps or online applications. Chatbots are conversational software. To emulate a human conversation, these conversational agents imitate human speech. Offering a customized and satisfying experience is of the utmost relevance for healthcare professionals as health services become more patient-centric.

Timing is crucial in the healthcare industry. Patients can obtain quick treatment at their fingertips with the aid of a medical chatbot. Chatbots are also crucial in an emergency situation, especially for older patients.

Practical applications:
- Voice assistants act as the first point of contact between the patient and the doctor.
- Many users prefer messaging than calling. On this front, chatbot's are exceptionally helpful. Currently, many healthcare systems use chatbot's to answer customer inquiries on websites and social media platforms like Facebook.

- With the help of chatbot, it is easy to track patient health record and analyze the data with a clinical application that helps the clinicians for diagnosis, treatment, and more.

AR and VR in healthcare: Technology advancements in healthcare are mostly made possible by AR and VR. The use of AR and VR in healthcare provides workable answers to a number of systemic problems and a wide range of options for deployment, including general diagnostics.

Visualizing patient data with the potential for real-time statistics is the simplest approach for augmented reality to integrate into the healthcare system. Patients who have ongoing medical conditions can keep an eye on them while relaxing in their own homes. A doctor can perform a virtual reality walkthrough to show the patient how to manage or quickly administer the medication if they require assistance. Additionally, AR is utilized to speed up certain processes, such the real-time overlay of patient information and vital signs on a doctor's examination of a patient.

Cloud computing: Instead than being a new technology, cloud computing is a new way to supply computer resources. Many healthcare institutions use cloud computing for their infrastructure management and administrative tasks. It provides the ability to communicate files, such as medical histories, billing information, and different therapies for improved healthcare administration.

Practical applications
- When a patient visits the healthcare institution, clinicians have access to information about the patient's medical history, allergies, the treatments provided, and several other crucial criteria.
- Medical experts and a patient located far can easily share information to provide an accurate diagnosis and treatment thanks to cloud computing.

Portal technology: The use of portal technology is one method that encourages patients to take an active role in their own healthcare. Medical professionals and patients can communicate online thanks to portal technology. With the help of this technology, patients can take a more active role in and learn more about their care. Portal technology can provide patients more control and accountability while also improving access to and availability of medical information. It is effective because a patient can function as an outstanding source and active participant in their treatment.

Blockchain and future healthcare technology: Accessibility, portability, and integrity of information in a complicated setting are issues that blockchain addresses. The loss or corruption of medical records kept in clinic databases is a constant possibility. Blockchain has the potential to upend the status quo, because it gives patients control over who can access their records. Who has access to the records and how they are utilized are both fully transparent.

When a patient is traveling to a different country, blockchain healthcare systems are effective. Without the patient needing to verbally supply the information, clinicians can quickly access medical records when a medical intervention is urgently required.

Introduction of artificial intelligence to data processing: The use of artificial intelligence is gaining popularity as it facilitates the automated manipulation of massive amounts of collected data to produce precise and quick results. Additionally, it aids in the extraction of crucial data from unstructured data, including text, photos, and videos. AI-based EMRs will be able to diagnose diseases more quickly by reducing the need for human intervention, which will enhance patient outcomes and lower costs associated with duplicative work and manual entry.

Robotic process automation: Because of enhanced workflow and increased accuracy, automated data capture is becoming more and more common in the electronic medical record market. Robotic automation (RPA) assists in achieving the requisite accuracy by doing away with the necessity for manual entry.

BENEFITS OF ELECTRONIC MEDICAL RECORDS

- **Accuracy:** Because manual data entry isn't involved, electronic medical records are quite accurate. It implies that there is no possibility of inaccurate or stale data being saved in the system. With no space for error, patients receive better care and have better outcomes.
- **Better governance:** In a system with a single point of access, medical professionals can view the patient's medical history, ensuring that they are informed of any previous treatments. Better data governance results in better macro and micro decision-making, which enhances patient care.
- **Convenient view:** Patients can easily access their medical records from any location and on any device at any time. It makes it simple to track information and makes it convenient for medical practitioners to review patient data.
- **Integration:** By integrating their electronic medical records (EMRs) with other systems including practise management software, ordering software for lab tests, imaging tools, and electronic health records (EHR), healthcare professionals can access aggregated patient data via a single interface. The procedure of providing patient care will be improved.
- **Better communication:** Using EMRs and HIPAA-compliant encrypted messaging apps, healthcare providers may connect with their patients more effectively. The EMR system saves these messages, adding an additional layer of protection for patients and healthcare personnel. These apps allow patients to text their doctors and get immediate responses.
- **Quicker transactions:** By processing insurance claim forms with pre-populated data entry sections, healthcare practitioners can save time and effort. It speeds up compensation and cuts down on pointless delays, which frequently cause patient care to be delayed. Additionally, billing software is included in EMRs, which eliminates errors brought on by human data entry by automatically calculating the billing codes for a certain treatment or diagnosis.

STANDARD FOR ELECTRONIC HEALTH RECORDS

The electronic health record (EHR) standards for India were notified by the Ministry of Health and Family Welfare (MoH FW) in September 2013. Keeping in mind their suitability for and applicability in India, the set of standards provided there were selected from the best accessible and utilized standards applicable to electronic health records from around the world. Experts, practitioners, government representatives, technologists, and representatives from business represented on the committee formed to recommend the standards. The declared standards were praised as a positive start in the right direction by a number of technical and social observers in addition to professional organizations, regulatory bodies, stakeholders, and stakeholders themselves.

Type	Standard Name	Intended Purpose
Identification and demographics	Health informatics–identification of subjects of healthcare	Basic identity details of patient
	Demographic (Person Identification and land region codification) version 1.1	Complete demographic for interoperability with E-Governance systems
Patient Identifiers	UIDAI Aadhaar	Preferable identifier where available
	Local Identifier	Identifier given within institution/clinic/lab
	Government issued photo identity card number	Identifier used in conjunction with local in absence of Aadhaar
Architecture Requirements	Health informatics–requirements for an electronic health record architecture	System architectural requirements
Functional Requirements	Health informatics–HL7 electronic health records-system functional model	System functional requirements
Reference Model and Composition	Health informatics–system of concepts to support continuity of care	Concepts for care, actors, activities, process, etc.
	Health informatics–electronic health record communication	Information model architecture and communication
Terminology	Clinical terms	Primary terminology
Coding System	Logical observation identifiers names and codes	Test, measurement, observations
	WHO family of international classifications	Classification and reporting
Imaging	Digital imaging and communications in medicine	Image, waveform, audio/video
Scanned or captured records	Coding of audio-visual objects	Audio/video capture format
Data exchange	Health informatics—electronic health record communication–part 5: interface specification	EHR archetypes exchange [Also, refer to openEHR Service Model specification]
	An application protocol for electronic data exchange in healthcare environments	Event/message exchange
Discharge/ treatment summary	Medical Council of India (MCI) under regulation 3.1 of ethics	Composition as prescribed
E-Prescription	Pharmacy practice regulations, 2015 Notification No. 14-148/ 2012- PCI as specified by Pharmacy Council of India	Composition as prescribed

SUMMARY

The best option right now for effective healthcare management is an EMR. In addition to speeding up decision-making and lowering expenses to make it affordable for all healthcare professionals, they provide reliable data gathering to ensure improved patient care. Future market growth for EMRs will be fueled by these factors. An electronic version of a patient's medical history, maintained over time by the healthcare provider, is known as an electronic health record (EHR). An EHR may contain all of the essential administrative clinical data relevant to that person's care under a specific provider, such as demographics, progress notes, issues, medications, vital signs, past medical histories, immunizations, laboratory results, and radiology reports. The EHR automates information access and has the potential to make the clinician's workflow more efficient. Through a variety of interfaces, the EHR can also directly or indirectly support other care-related activities, such as quality control, outcomes reporting, and evidence-based decision support.

REVIEW QUESTION

1. What is electronic health records? What are the challenges in implementing the EHR system in nursing?
2. How electronic health record system helps nursing services to give optimal patient care?
3. What are the latest trends in electronic health record system?
4. How to implement electronic health record system in nursing services?
5. What are the key components of electronic health record system? Explain any three.

MULTIPLE CHOICE QUESTIONS

1. **What was the driving force behind the requirement for electronic health records (EHRs)?**
    a. The expansion of the health insurance market
    b. Better medical care for patients
    c. Improving the working environment for medical professionals
    d. The development of computer science

2. **What information is more available to doctors because of the inception of EHRs?**
    a. Drug dosages
    b. Side effects
    c. Allergies
    d. All of these

3. **What is one advanced method used to input data into an EHR?**
    a. Using a keyboard to type
    b. Play your iPod
    c. Employ voice recognition technology
    d. Making use of a transcriber

4. **Which of the following features is not a positive attribute of EHRs?**
    a. Enhanced accessibility to clinical information
    b. Improved client safety
    c. Increased quality of client care
    d. Decreased efficiency and savings

Shared Care and Electronic Health Records

5. **What technology advancement has made it easier for medical workers to move around?**
   a. Handheld computers
   b. Wireless connectivity
   c. PDAs
   d. All of these

6. **Which of the following is a barrier to the implementation of EHR?**
   a. Lack of standards
   b. E-prescribing options
   c. Identified ROI
   d. Increased patient safety

7. **Which technological advancements have made it easier to access medical databases over long distances?**
   a. Internet
   b. LANs
   c. Smart phones
   d. None of these

8. **When might internet technologies benefit a healthcare provider?**
   a. Whenever they use a hospital's EHR
   b. When using a nursing home to access their EHR
   c. When using a home office to access their EHR
   d. All of these

9. **Which of the following is not a benefit of EHR?**
   a. Little or no training necessary
   b. Enhanced access to clinical information
   c. Improved patient safety
   d. Decreased medical errors

Answer Key

1. b
2. d
3. d
4. d
5. d
6. b
7. a
8. d
9. a

CHAPTER 5

Patient Safety and Clinical Risk

At the end of this chapter, student will able to learn about:
- Patient safety
- Purposes of patient safety informatics
- Methods of patient safety informatics
- Risk management process
- Process of risk management process
- Importance of risk management process

TERMINOLOGIES

- **Patient safety:** It is a branch of medicine that came into being as healthcare systems became more complicated and patient harm in medical facilities increased as a result. (WHO)
- **Patient safety informatics:** It is the process of gathering, analyzing, and managing health data, as well as the use of medical principles in conjunction with health IT systems to ensure safe treatment and enable physicians to make better decisions.
- **Risk:** Anything that has the potential to cause an unanticipated consequence or a loss.
- **Risk management:** It is the process of analyzing current processes and practises, identifying risk factors, and putting policies in place to handle those risks.
- **Enterprise risk management:** In the healthcare industry encourages a thorough framework for risk management decisions that maximize value protection and production by managing risk and uncertainty and their relationships to total value.
- **Risk mitigation:** It involves analyzing the likelihood that a positive or negative event will occur that has an impact as well as the interventions to lessen the negative consequence.
- **Risk management process:** The process of detecting, monitoring, and managing possible risks in order to reduce any negative effects they may have on a company is known as risk management. Examples include data loss, system malfunctions, and security breaches.

PATIENT SAFETY AND INFORMATICS

Introduction

HISs prioritize safety above all else. In order to assist healthcare professionals in giving patients safe and effective medical care, HISs must operate accurately, steadily, and smoothly. Additionally, patient data must be stored properly and securely. "Safety" is broken down into a variety of categories in the HIS context, some of which are regulated by law. One of these categories is "patient safety," which relates to the idea that HISs will help prevent medical mishaps like patient mistakes (such as doing surgery in the wrong place) and issues with drug delivery. In reality, hospitals with actively customized HISs have built features that promote patient safety by collaborating with contracted suppliers and utilizing incident report analysis from the institutions themselves.

Patient safety is one of the most important "safety" obligations that HISs is expected to fulfiil. Along with the expansion of HISs, patient safety concerns have increased, and patient safety advancement programmes have also gained in popularity. In order to address the issue of patient safety, the majority of large hospitals place a high priority on the health of their patients. However, there was no proof connecting HIS to a decrease in unfavorable outcomes brought on by medical intervention.

METHODS USED IN HOSPITAL INFORMATION SYSTEM FOR PATIENT SAFETY

- Internal medicine prescriptions written for one dose (printing with the daily dose)
- Using master files consistently in systems for obtaining prescription drugs
- Recognizing high-risk substances and controlling them with system help
- The overdose check and alarm feature
- Checking and alerting for dosing contraindications
- A feature for printing the constituent amounts for a prescription drug
- Off-label medication screening and alarm feature
- Interaction/drug check/alert functionality that is contraindicated
- A feature for comparing prescriptions from several clinical departments for consistency
- Preventative actions to avoid choosing incorrect medications with similar names (three-character input, etc.)
- Checking the accuracy of drug orders and drug allergy information
- Checking that meal orders and information about food allergies
- Calendar-format display function
- Management and prescription system for medicines taken by patients
- Information about allergies is transferred from the main system to departmental systems
  - Compatibility with the pharmacy department
  - Integration with the department of radiation
  - Including the endoscopy department in the process
  - Integration with the department of nutrition-management
- **Introduction of new systems (equipment) and functions: The addition of safety functions**
  - A feature for preventing patients from registering more than once electronic clinical paths are introduced
  - Development of a mechanism to monitor chemotherapy regimens

- Notification of aberrant test results to the attending physician (the doctor who issues instructions)
- Notification of unread pathology/imaging test results to the attending doctor (the doctor who issues orders)
- The ability to send implant-related confirmation messages prior to MRIs
- Ability to check blood type while placing an order for blood transfusions
- A feature that records a patient's blood type
- Checking whether a patient's blood type matches the plasma type while ordering plasma products
- Blood transfusion/biopharmaceutical traceability and of biological and medical materials

Frameworks Used by Organizations for Patient Safety Outcomes Through Informatics

- **Health information governance:** Organizations must establish a health information oversight mechanism that includes leadership and relevant stakeholders. In addition, organizations need to ensure that their health information plan is coordinated with the organization's patient safety and risk management plan.
- **Safety risk identification:** Organizations need to identify areas that health information technology might aid in improving patient safety namely, medication safety, guideline adherence, and so forth.
- **Stakeholder involvement:** Stakeholders need to be involved in all phases of health information projects from planning and implementation until continuous improvement. The most important stakeholder must be the system end-user and process owner.
- **Informed decision:** Organizations need to review the cost effectiveness of suggested technologies, which includes conducting an evidence based decision and an evaluation of the current information technology infrastructure including software and hardware.
- **Sufficient training:** Organizations need to ensure that all relevant line staff receive sufficient training on the use of the proposed health information technology.
- **Gradual implementation:** Rolling out the technology in a gradual stepped approach is crucial to avoid disruption of current processes and systems.
- **Continuous evaluation and monitoring of patient safety outcomes:** Organizations need to measure patient safety outcomes on a continuous basis especially during the initial implementation to ensure that the new technology achieves its intended outcome.
- **Technology optimization:** Organizations need to modify and finetune the implemented technology based on user feedback and patient safety outcomes.
- **Regular technology updates:** Organizations must ensure that health information technologies are continuously updated to comply with recent best clinical practices, regulatory standards, and technical stability.

INFORMATION TECHNOLOGY WITH THE GREATEST IMPACT ON PATIENT SAFETY

Even though each medical procedure has unique requirements, the following are the areas where health IT has so far had the most influence on patient safety.

Easy Information Access

Health IT specialists have been working on interoperability—the capacity to transfer patient data across various systems—for years. As digital systems develop in this field, practitioners are able to share patient information, reducing the possibility of treating a patient incorrectly. For instance, a doctor at a hospital has access to a patient's medical records through their personal doctor. It can also be helpful in warning medical professionals when a pandemic first emerges, as the COVID-19 emergency has shown.

Adoption of Electronic Health Records

The work responsibilities of nurses and other staff members have been significantly impacted by electronic medical records and electronic health records. Nurses now need to know how to enter patient data into the system. The appropriate codes are updated in the records by medical coders. These documents are also used by the billing division to submit insurance claims. Overall, the care patients receive is better and more effective thanks to digitized medical records.

Reduction of Drug-related Errors

Drug prescription errors are medical mistakes that could have devastating effects. Errors in this area have been reduced with the use of electronic prescribing. By converting handwritten prescriptions to electronic entry on a secure device, automatically checking for drug interactions, automating requests for refills and reminders, and raising warnings in the event of a suspected medication error, these systems lessen the possibility of medication errors.

Improved Public Health

Public health entails recognising chronic health problems within particular population demographics and developing preventive initiatives that help individuals stay healthy for longer. Public health informatics, which focuses on the entire population, uses data from numerous sources, including hospitals, social services, surveys, and more, to assist healthcare practitioners and governmental organizations in addressing and preparing for emerging health concerns.

For instance, EHR data is highly important when using analytics for public health management since it enables researchers to identify issues earlier (like a flu outbreak) and take faster action (in the case of flu, getting more vaccines into the affected community).

Support for Clinical Decisions

One of the most important areas where technology may increase patient safety is clinical decision support (CDS). Utilizing technology, CDS includes putting all pertinent data about a patient and defined guidelines on prospective therapies in the hands of a doctor in real-time.

AHRQ reports that a study using CDS in oncology treatment discovered "enhanced clinical practise guideline use and concordance, improved care process measures, and reduced safety incidents."

FUTURE OF INFORMATION TECHNOLOGY AND PATIENT SAFETY

Healthcare is one of many sectors where applications for artificial intelligence (AI) and machine learning have yet to be fully realized. AHRQ indicated that CDS can be expanded and improved by AI in the same paper. According to the paper, contemporary AI systems can, for instance, identify warning indications of patient deterioration or complex illnesses like sepsis.

The business of healthcare can also benefit from the use of AI and machine learning. Many of the repetitive billing and coding tasks can be handled by advanced technologies, freeing up humans to undertake more difficult tasks.

Predictive health analytics is a different field that has grown in popularity recently.

RISK MANAGEMENT PROCESS

Introduction

Risk is something that carries a chance of an unanticipated result or a loss. Risk can be found in practically every area, including the financial sector, transportation, and even the health care sector. Even if there is no way to completely eliminate risk, there is a technique to manage it risk management. By diversifying your investments and redistributing the assets in your investment portfolio, you can reduce your risks in the financial sector. Through innovation and development, businesses may be able to control their risks. But how does this operate in the medical field?

The stakes are even higher in healthcare since risk management might mean the difference between life and death. Risk management in the healthcare sector may be more crucial than in any other sector in several ways. Risks in the healthcare industry include medical misconduct, treatments, defective equipment, and other hazards. To keep people secure and safe and to control costs, the healthcare sector must effectively manage these and other risks. Hospitals, long-term care institutions, and other healthcare organizations can reduce the possibility of loss once risk management methods are in place.

Definition

- The process of identifying specific risk areas, creating a detailed plan, integrating the plan, and carrying out ongoing evaluations is known as risk management.
- Insuring against losses, safeguarding investments from interest rate drops, and hedging loans against rate increases are all examples of risk management techniques.
- The clinical and administrative systems, processes, and reports used in risk management in the healthcare industry include those for risk detection, monitoring, assessment, mitigation, and prevention. Healthcare organizations that use risk management proactively and methodically protect patient safety as well as their assets, market share, accreditation, levels of reimbursement, brand value, and reputation in the community.
- Healthcare risk management aids in defending healthcare organizations against a variety of threats unique to the sector. For instance, they avoid issues with administrative systems, patient data, and more.

IMPORTANCE OF RISK MANAGEMENT IN HEALTHCARE

Risk management is crucial in the healthcare sector for numerous reasons. The main advantages of a healthcare risk management solution are listed and along with some of the issues they assist avoid.

- **Improve patient safety:** Protecting patient records is the most crucial part of risk management in healthcare. The Health Insurance Portability and Accountability Act, or HIPAA, stipulates that all medical information must be kept private. This data needs to be kept secure. A healthcare institution may experience several problems if HIPAA laws are broken. Some forms of risk management in healthcare focus on privacy laws, prevent data breaches, and guarantee that patient information is kept private.
- **Data security:** Data security is essential to protect patient information, as was previously stated. However, cyberattacks and other issues that result in data leaks are a prevalent issue in the modern world. Your company's ability to respond quickly to problems will be enhanced if you have a risk management strategy in place and are ready for these potential outcomes.
- **Plan for catastrophes:** Having a risk management strategy also makes it much easier to prepare for disasters. When you work in healthcare, you never know when an emergency may arise. These can include things like data leaks and natural disasters. Disease outbreaks are another frequent sort of emergency in the healthcare sector. It is crucial to have a strategy in place for when these types of outbreaks occur, especially if you work in a hospital. This will not only expedite the problem-solving process but also safeguard your patients. Plans for risk management assist you in properly responding to and reporting on any disasters you may encounter.
- **Effective patient care practices:** Healthcare risk management plans are created and put into action based on in-depth, continuing research. Healthcare risk managers must stay current on pertinent knowledge in their industry because study findings may contradict assumptions that would otherwise guide risk management procedures. One study, for instance, found that increasing the amount of sleep that residents in teaching hospitals got actually made patient safety less safe. The goal of risk management was to make sure that measures were taken to improve resident sleep patterns and lower patient risks.

STEPS IN RISK MANAGEMENT PROCESS

A five-step management decision-making model is used in the risk management process. Below are listed the first five fundamental steps in risk management **(Fig. 5.1)**.

Five Basic Steps of Risk Management

Step 1: Establishing the context is the first step in managing and identifying risks. The context-sensitively high priority areas for risk management in connection to patient care are the intensive care unit, operating room, medication management, including drug delivery.

Step 2: The process by which healthcare professionals and staff members become aware of the hazards in the environment and services related to healthcare is known as risk identification. The risks found are put in the Risk Management Tool (RMT), sometimes referred to as the Risk Register.

Sources of Risk Identification
- Conversations with department heads, managers, and employees
- Activity tracked by the patient (Tracing the journey of a patient from admission till discharge)

❐ Examining patient records in the past
❐ Accreditation body reports
❐ Sentinel events and incident reporting system
❐ Reports on healthcare-associated illnesses
❐ Reports from the executive committee
❐ Report from the facility management and safety committee
❐ Survey findings on patient complaints and satisfaction

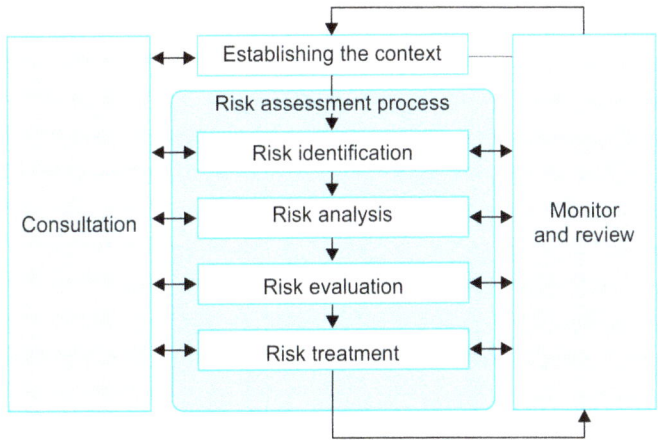

Fig. 5.1: Risk management process.

Step 3: Analyze risks: Understanding the risk that has been discovered is the goal of risk analysis. It consists of the following: Risk levels or scores, underlying causes, already in place controls. Root Cause Analysis (RCA) is a methodical way to determining the root causes of unfavourable events so that appropriate action can be done to change procedures and stop such losses. The most effective way to conduct root cause analysis is still to brainstorm with a group of pertinent and knowledgeable individuals. Various risk assessment healthcare tools can be utilized as shown in **Figures 5.2 and 5.3**.

Step 4: Assess the risks: The goals of risk assessment are to decide which hazards need to be treated and how to treat them based on the results of the risk analysis.

Step 5A: Treating the risk (also known as reducing the risk or mitigating the risk): Decisions about risk management should be made while taking into account the objectives and goals of the service as well as the stated internal, external, and risk management settings. A risk management strategy should:
❐ Proposed actions
❐ Resource requirements
❐ Persons responsible for actions
❐ Time frames

Step 5B: Controlling the risk: The best risk management practises involve redesigning the systems and procedures to lessen the likelihood of a negative event. Reducing the risk's likelihood and/or the impact's severity are two more strategies for risk management.

Risk management tool in healthcare

Department: _____

System/process: _____

1-5	Low risk
5-25	Medium risk
25-45	High risk

Risk identified	Date risk identified	Causes	Current controls in the system	Likelihood (L) (score 1 to 5)	Impact severity (S) (Score 1 to 5)	Overall risk rating R= L×S (High, Medium, Low)	Risk response strategy (Accept, control, transfer, avoid)	Actions required	Responsible person/s	Resources required	Due date for actions	Post treatment likelihood (L) score 1 to 5	Post treatment impact severity (S) score 1 to 5	Post-treatment risk score (High, medium, low)	Review date	Contingency plan (What will you do if the risk really happens?)
				4	5	20						1	4	4		
						0								0		
						0								0		
						0								0		
						0								0		
						0								0		
						0								0		
						0								0		
						0								0		
						0								0		
						0								0		

Fig. 5.2: Risk management register.

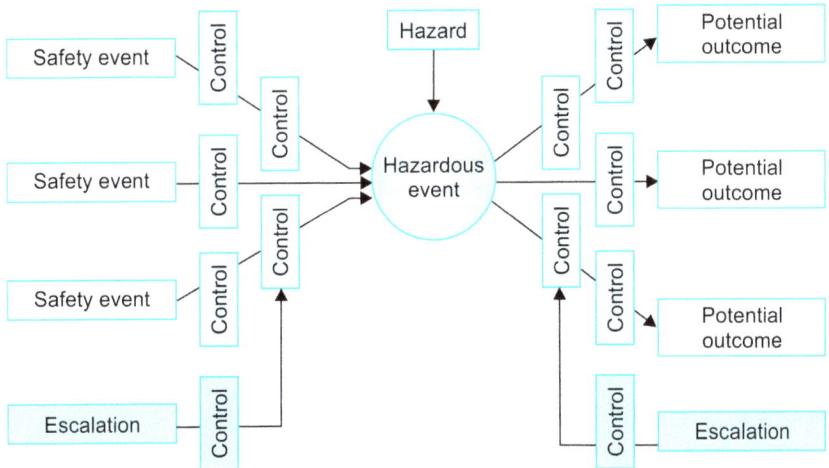

Fig. 5.3: Bowtie model as risk assessment tool.

APPLICATIONS OF RISK MANAGEMENT PROCESS

Identification of Risk

Using checklists of potential hazards and assessing the possibility that those events could occur on the project are part of a more disciplined approach. Based on knowledge gained from previous projects, certain businesses and sectors created risk checklists. The project manager and project team can use these checklists to identify specific risks on the list and to broaden the team's perspective. Project team members' prior experiences, company-wide project experience, and industry specialists can all be useful resources for spotting possible risks on a project **(Fig. 5.4)**.

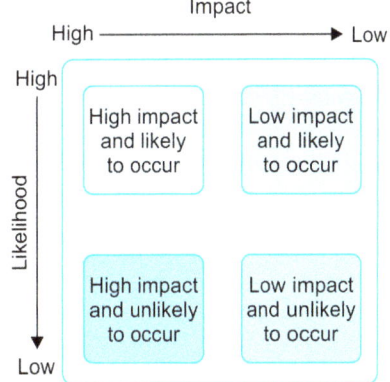

Fig. 5.4: Risk matrix model.

Risk Assessment

The project team assessees each potential risk after it has been identified, taking into account both the likelihood that the risk event will occur and any potential losses that could result from it. Risks are not created equal. Risk occurrences can cost a wide range of amounts and some are more likely to occur than others. The following phase in the risk management process involves assessing the risk for likelihood of occurrence and severity, or the potential loss to the project.

Risk Reduction

The project team creates a risk mitigation plan, which is a strategy to lessen the effects of an unexpected event, after the risk has been recognized and assessed.
- Risk reduction
- Sharing of risk
- Risk mitigation
- Risk shifting

Each of these risk-mitigation strategies has the potential to be a powerful instrument for lowering both individual hazards and the project's overall risk profile. Each identified risk event's risk mitigation strategy and the steps the project management team will take to minimize or eliminate the risk are documented in the risk mitigation plan **(Fig. 5.4)**.

Risk avoidance: It often entails creating an alternative plan of action with a higher chance of success but typically a higher cost to complete a project assignment. Utilizing tried-and-true technologies rather than adopting novel ones, despite the latter's potential for superior performance or lower costs, is a popular risk avoidance strategy. To avoid the risk of working with a new vendor, a project team may opt for a vendor with a track record of success versus a new vendor offering considerable price incentives. By requiring drug testing for team members, the project team is reducing risk by preventing harm from being done by someone under the influence of drugs.

Risk sharing: It entails working together with others to split the burden of the risky activity. By forming a joint venture with a company based in another country, many organizations that work on international projects can lessen the political, legal, labour, and other risk types involved with such initiatives. When the other organization possesses knowledge and experience the project team lacks, partnering with them to share the risk associated with a portion of the project is useful. The partnering company takes on some or all of the unfavorable effects of the risk event, if it does occur. Additionally, a portion of the earnings or benefit from a successful project will go to the company.

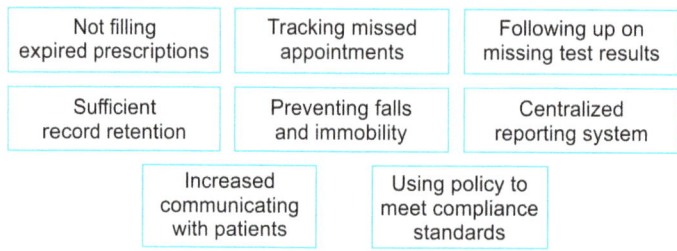

Fig. 5.5: Ways to manage risk in healthcare.

SUMMARY

Patient safety is a healthcare discipline that arose as a consequence of the increasing complexity of health care systems and the increase in patient harm in healthcare institutions. Its goal is to avoid and decrease risks, mistakes, and damage to patients while providing healthcare. Continuous improvement based on learning from mistakes and bad occurrences is a cornerstone of the profession.

Patient safety is critical to providing high-quality vital health services. Indeed, there is broad agreement that great healthcare should be effective, safe, and people-centered across the globe. Furthermore, for the advantages of excellent healthcare to be realized, health services must be timely, equitable, integrated, and efficient.

Clear policies, leadership ability, data to drive safety improvements, experienced healthcare personnel, and effective patient engagement in their care are all required to enable the successful implementation of patient safety programmes.

Patient Safety and Clinical Risk

REVIEW QUESTION

1. Define patient safety informatics.
2. Decribe risk management process.
3. Discuss the process of risk management process.
4. Discuss the importance of risk management process.
5. Define patient safety.
6. Discuss briefly IT framework used by organizations for patient safety.
7. How technology assist in clinical decision support in patient safety?
8. What is artificial intelligence?
9. Define risk management.
10. What is enterprise risk management?
11. Discuss, in detail, about patient safety informatics.
12. Discuss the impact of information technology on patient safety.
13. Discuss the applications of risk management process.
14. Elaborate the importance of risk management process in healthcare.

MULTIPLE CHOICE QUESTIONS

1. **Nursing informatics plays a vital role in keeping patients safe through technology. In what part of patient care does patient safety play a role?**
   a. Patient safety is important while the patient is receiving care after surgery.
   b. Patient safety is important in the transfer of patients room one department to another.
   c. Patient safety is important in the procedure or operating room, recovery room, and transfer back to the unit.
   d. Patient safety is important from the first contact with the patient through care after discharge.

2. **Many nurses, along with software developers, are creating patient safety features for the electronic medical record. Which of these is a common safety feature?**
   a. Scanning bar codes on medication and patient armbands
   b. Allergy alerts for medication
   c. Hard stops for all staff to fill out vital information at critical junctures such as blood transfusions
   d. All of the answers are correct

3. **Equipment-related accidents are risks in the healthcare agency. The nurse assessees for this risk when using**
   a. Sequential compression devices
   b. A measuring device that measures urine
   c. Computer-based documentation
   d. A manual medication-dispensing device

4. **Which of these safety measures should be a standard procedure for hospital doctors and nurses?**
   a. Washing hands before treating a patient
   b. Checking the patient's ID bracelet before giving any medicine
   c. Thoroughly explaining the reasons for any test or treatment
   d. All of the above

5. **Risk management is the most important process to be handled by:**
   a. Client
   b. Investor
   c. Production team
   d. Project manager

6. Which of the following risk are derived from hardware or software technologies that are used to develop the system?
   a. Managerial risk
   b. Technological risk
   c. Estimation risk
   d. Organizational risk

7. Risk management can be defined as the art and science of _____ risk factors throughout the life cycle of a project.
   a. Researching, reviewing, and acting on
   b. Identifying, analyzing, and responding to
   c. Reviewing, monitoring, and managing
   d. Identifying, reviewing, and avoiding
   e. Analyzing, changing, and suppressing

8. Risk management includes all of the following processes, *except*:
   a. Risk monitoring and control
   b. Risk identification
   c. Risk avoidance
   d. Risk response planning
   e. Risk management planning

9. Risk mitigation involves all but which of the following:
   a. Developing system standards (policies, procedures, responsibility standards)
   b. Obtaining insurance against loss
   c. Identification of project risks
   d. Performing contingent planning
   e. Developing planning alternatives

Answer Key

1. d
2. d
3. c
4. d
5. d
6. b
7. a
8. c
9. c

CHAPTER 6

Clinical Knowledge and Decision Making

At the end of this chapter, student will able to learn about:

- Knowledge management system
- Dimensions of knowledge management system
- Components of knowledge management system
- Advantages of knowledge management system
- Challenges of knowledge management system
- Importance of knowledge management in healthcare and clinical
- Knowledge management methods (Advantages and disadvantages)
- Standards in health informatics
- Systematized nomenclature of medicine—clinical terms (SNOMED-CT)
- Applications of SNOMED-CT

TERMINOLOGIES

- **Communities of practise (CoP):** Groups of people who work on related tasks or in related fields who get together to share knowledge and advance their professions for the benefit of their organizations and themselves (s). They can be developed formally or informally, and they can communicate in person or online.
- **CBT stands for computer-based training:** CBT refers to interactive computers used to offer training. Modern CBT may feature embedded intelligence to help students or challenge them, multimedia (sounds, video clips), and hyper-links. Some CBT let students respond to simulated real-life scenarios (like dealing with an irate customer) and record their conduct as the computer modifies the course of the engagement.
- **Customer relationship management (CRM):** It is a business strategy that focuses on identifying and actively managing the most important customer connections. Effective marketing, sales, and customer service procedures demand a customer-focused mentality.
- **Encoding** is the process of converting data into a format required for a number of information.

INTRODUCTION

Compared to the animal realm, human knowledge transfer is significantly more broad and complicated. Perhaps the most common method for sharing knowledge is through human language. Early on in the history of humanity, nomadic tribes brought their traditions, practises, and—most importantly—their technology to many different regions of the globe. The first masters of knowledge transfer were the villagers' storytellers, who would recite tales verbatim while imparting lessons from earlier generations. The written word improved language; the printing press and later technological instruments improved the written word. There are still basic issues with information transfer, notwithstanding technical advancements. In today's knowledge economy, the capacity to handle knowledge is essential.

The production and dissemination of information have grown in significance as competitiveness-enhancing elements. Knowledge is increasingly regarded as a precious resource that is contained in goods (especially high-tech goods) and contained in the tacit knowledge of employees who move about a lot. Despite the fact that information is increasingly seen as a commodity or intellectual asset, it has several contradictory qualities that distinguish it apart from other valued commodities.

KNOWLEDGE MANAGEMENT SYSTEM

Any IT system that saves and retrieves knowledge to enhance comprehension, teamwork, and process alignment is referred to as a knowledge management system. Knowledge management systems can be used to organize your knowledge base for your users or customers as well as among companies or teams.

The systematic administration of an organization's knowledge assets for the purpose of adding value and satisfying tactical and strategic requirements is known as knowledge management. It consists of the programmes, procedures, plans, and mechanisms that support and improve the gathering, evaluating, sharing, and creation of knowledge.

Knowledge management should be outlined in terms of the individual business goals of each organization. Applying information to new, previously burdened, or unique situations is the core of knowledge management.

Dimensions of Knowledge Management System

It's crucial to keep in mind that managing knowledge isn't about managing knowledge for knowledge's sake. The overarching purpose is to add value while utilizing, enhancing, and improving the firm's knowledge assets to achieve organizational goals.

Thus, there are several aspects to knowledge management implementation, such as:
- **Strategy:** The corporate strategy must inform the knowledge management strategy. Managing, distributing, and producing pertinent knowledge assets that support tactical and strategic goals is the goal.
- **Organizational culture:** An organization's culture affects how people interact, the environment in which knowledge is produced, their willingness to accept change, and ultimately, how they share information (or do not share it).
- **Organizational processes:** The ideal procedures, surroundings, and frameworks that permit KM implementation within the company.
- **Management and leadership:** All levels of KM require professional and seasoned leadership. An organization may or may not need to implement a range of KM-related positions, such as a CKO, knowledge managers, knowledge brokers, and so forth. The section on KM positions and duties has more information on this.
- **Technology:** The systems, tools, and technologies that are appropriately planned and put into place to meet the needs of the organization.

☐ **Politics:** The long-term support for programmes that encompass almost all organizational activities, may be expensive to accomplish (both in terms of time and money), and frequently do not immediately show a return on investment.

Components of Knowledge Management System

Knowledge management is currently seen as a continuous cycle of four processes:

Knowledge of Discovery

Knowledge needs to be discovered before being put to use! Knowledge discovery refers to developing new tacit and explicit knowledge from raw data. We must refine raw data to generate valuable information and then analyze and process it into knowledge.

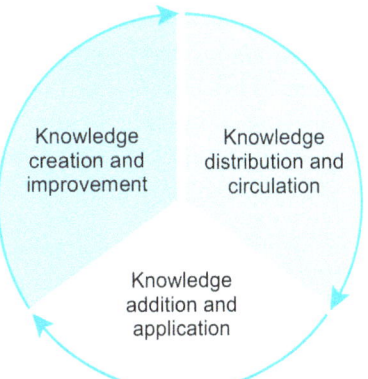

Fig. 6.1: Components of KMS (Kindly add all 4 components).

Examples of processes commonly used for knowledge discovery are surveys, questionnaires, individual interviews, group interviews, and observation.

Knowledge discovery, the first step of the knowledge management process involves communication, integration, and systemization of multiple streams of explicit knowledge. Tacit knowledge is implied knowledge that is discovered by socialization, for example, through joint activities, instead of written or oral instructions.

Knowledge of Capture

Knowledge capture is the part of knowledge management process that deals with retrieving explicit or tacit knowledge that resides within people, artifacts, or organizational entities.

Tacit knowledge is captured from the employees through externalization, which involves documentation, verbalization, and sharing; for example, forming quality circles to improve a specific business process.

Internalization, another process of knowledge management, involves the acquiring of tacit knowledge by employees through learning. Additionally, internalization is the process of converting the employee's tacit knowledge into explicit by applying it to practical situations. For example, organizations conduct on-job training or practical training sessions for the employees through simulation or experiments.

Knowledge of Sharing

The organization now has a considerable chunk of explicit or tacit knowledge. But, it is a waste if they cannot share it across for use. As it is said, knowledge shared is knowledge squared!

So, knowledge sharing is the process of making the relevant explicit or tacit knowledge available to the right people at the right time. Knowledge sharing additionally benefits businesses by improving communication among team members.

For example, knowledge sharing involves writing books, research papers, delivering a speech, lectures, presentations, training events, forums. Technology has enabled organizations to have shared project files where multiple team members can work together and contribute to managing knowledge sharing effectively.

Knowledge of Application

Last but not least, the knowledge discovered, captured, and shared has to be applied for the benefit of the business. All the efforts in the process of knowledge management fail if this application or implementation is not effective.

Knowledge application is about the actualization of knowledge to make decisions, improve processes, and make the best use of this knowledge to solve business problems. The essential knowledge chunks are leveraged to make business decisions. Knowledge is also applied organization-wide through instructions, procedures, norms, etc.

Knowledge application has become more comfortable these days with the help of technology. For example, numerous business intelligence tools like SAP business intelligence leverage Artificial Intelligence (AI) and Machine Learning (ML) to process the knowledge data and offer analytics and reporting for better decision making.

Advantages of Knowledge Management System

- Supported employee growth and development
- Shared specialist expertise
- Better communication
- Better business processes
- Better decision-making
- Quicker problem-solving
- Quicker innovation
- Improved organizational agility
- Better and faster decision-making
- Better products and services
- Improve profitability, reuse existing knowledge and skills, create better plans, boost operational effectiveness, and boost employee output
- Early market trend recognition will provide you an advantage over your competitors
- Compare yourself to your rivals and maximise your group's collective intellectual capital

Challenges of Knowledge Management System

Knowing your limitations is essential for any knowledge management system to succeed. Some of the typical difficulties include:
- Making it easier to find information and resources
- Encouraging people to share, reuse, and apply knowledge consistently
- Aligning knowledge management with overall goals and business strategy
- Choosing and implementing knowledge management technology
- Integrating knowledge management into current processes and information systems
- Finding effective ways to capture and record business knowledge

Importance of Knowledge Management in Healthcare and Clinical

The ecology of healthcare is built on data. Informed decision-making, improved medical results, and seamless communication among healthcare professionals are all benefits of effective data management in the industry.
- **Powers accurate medical decisions:** It has the ability to make accurate medical decisions. Even the smallest mistake made by a healthcare worker can result in a patient losing their life. A single error could result in a catastrophe and a lawsuit. Healthcare knowledge

management gives doctors and nurses 24/7 consolidated access to patient-specific data and the most recent scientific findings to aid in making well-informed decisions.
- **Encourages a learning-focused environment:** Healthcare professionals cannot solely rely on the knowledge they acquired in medical school because the healthcare sector is growing quickly. To deliver top-notch services, they must stay current on the newest medical techniques, technology, and pharmacological advancements. Because of this, a number of international healthcare organizations mandate that practitioners obtain continuing education credits at least twice a year. In this quest, a knowledge management system can be useful.
- **Provides patients with self-help resources:** Patients anticipate having easy access to their medical records after registering with a hospital. They should be informed of their illness' current state and any recent developments. A healthcare knowledge management system makes sure that patients don't have to search far and wide for the information they need. They can use your patient site to log their interactions with doctors and keep tabs on the course of their treatments.
- **Upholds secrecy:** In the healthcare industry, maintaining confidentiality is required by ethical standards. Identity theft and data-related fraud are on the rise, and security breaches pose a serious threat to patients' lives. This can be avoided with a robust healthcare knowledge management system.
- **Avoid malpractice:** Medical malpractice is costly in more ways than one. An institutionalized knowledge management system of new findings and firsthand experiences will empower healthcare providers to partake in knowledge sharing in a way that's never been done before. This level of access to health informatics and information management systems would cut down on fatal misdiagnoses and ultimately streamline medical decision-making and improve the efficacy of nursing intervention.
- **Valuable results:** The goal of work is to deliver worthwhile results. Applied knowledge produces worthwhile outcomes. For effectiveness, heightened collaboration, and increased competition, organizational knowledge is emerging as a critical differentiator. The goal of work is to deliver worthwhile results. Applied knowledge produces worthwhile outcomes. For effectiveness, heightened collaboration, and increased competition, organizational knowledge is emerging as a critical differentiator.
- The importance of knowledge labour is rising in many communities and organizations. Knowledge is the primary source of prosperity in knowledge economies, which are what many economies strive to be. Knowledge becomes a key resource for enterprises in this situation. Knowledge is crucial for many reasons, including decision-making effectiveness, process efficiency support and improvement, resilience and adaptability creation, competitive advantage creation, and even the potential to become a product unto itself. An increased access to knowledge will create opportunities for the professional development of people in the organization through learning, practices and exchanges.
- To keep up with the rate of change, organizations can no longer rely on the natural spread of knowledge. Instead, knowledge needs to be consciously developed, consolidated, used, and reused at a higher rate than change.
- Sharing best practises, knowledge, and knowledge across organizational boundaries can greatly benefit geographically scattered and decentralized firms that carry out the same processes and provide the same services in many locations. Workforce attrition and turnover in today's society has implications for knowledge management. In many organizations,

critical knowledge is often retained by experts, at the risk of being lost when the organization changes or these experts leave.
- Effective knowledge management supports collaboration between different organizations to achieve shared objectives.

KNOWLEDGE MANAGEMENT METHODS

The structure of a company's knowledge management will vary depending on its needs. Common examples of information management techniques in use are shown below:
- **Tutoring and training:** Directly disseminating knowledge from the knowledge owner to other employees. This could be accomplished through in-person coaching, corporate training events, internet conversations, and focus groups. For improved training purposes, senior nurses or academicians in the field of nursing education might mentor the staff or junior nurses.

  Advantages
  - In-person learning tends to be more memorable.
  - Questions can be answered right away.
  - Clarifications can be given if the content is not understood.
  - Brainstorming sessions may be enabled.
  - Questions can be asked right away.

  Disadvantages
  - It can be time-consuming and distract from the tasks the knowledge holder is trying to complete.
  - It can take time to create and maintain a system of expertise location.
  - It can be difficult to document and save for later use.
  - It can be challenging to find the right expert with good communication skills and knowledge of the business.

- **Documentations, guides, guidelines:** Written communication is excellent for knowledge storage and transfer. A mechanism to store, categorise, and navigate topics is always available with text-based knowledge management.

  Advantages:
  - The organization has a useful source of current information.
  - Information is simple to access and distribute online.
  - It is simple to combine the experience of various people into one packet.

  Disadvantages:
  - It takes a lot of time to generate and keep current.
  - It needs to be managed properly to guarantee that pertinent information is easily accessed.
  - It needs infrastructure; and it takes time to use.

- **Forums, intranets, and collaboration environments:** These internet sites encourage discussion and gather lots of experts in one location. It is possible to categorize threads, subforums, and groups according to topic, level of competence, or a variety of other factors.

  Advantages:
  - Innovation is fueled by cooperation.
  - No matter where they are in the world, many specialists can congregate in one spot.
  - Facilitating communication with distant teams promotes teamwork and knowledge sharing.

  Disadvantages:
  - While information is submitted to discussions
  - It is not actively verified. It takes time to search through several messages and threads for pertinent replies.
  - Messages and threads may not be archived.

Clinical Knowledge and Decision Making

- **Learning and development environments:** Employees will continually seek out education if they work in a culture where it is valued. By rewarding them for using your knowledge management systems, you may upskill your workforce and prepare them for leadership positions in your company.
  Advantages:
  - Wide range of resources are available to create a constant flow of new content.
  - The structure facilitates easier subject discovery.
  - Authoring tools are available so that internal experts can create company-specific courses.
  - Analytical tools are available to help identify knowledge gaps within the organization.
  - Motivated employees can develop themselves at will; training pathways can be laid out.
  - Wide range of resources are available to produce a constant flow of fresh content.
  Disadvantages:
  - It requires a lot of effort to develop and maintain in house.
  - It readily available solutions may be too generic to add real value for your company.
  - Content must be created and continually updated.
  - Requires an influential learning culture to motivate staff to participate.
- **Case studies**: These in-depth studies into particular areas serve as complete guides to a subject. Looking at the actions taken, the results they produce, and any lessons learned are extremely valuable.
  Advantages:
  - Allow for complete documentation and archiving of lessons learned
  - Easily shareable
  - Efficient for communicating complex information
  Disadvantages:
  - It takes a lot of time and skill to create.
  - The case study may have limitations or require approval from the parties involved.
  - It can be too specialized to apply the knowledge broadly.
- **Webinars:** These online seminars can be beneficial in widely disseminating ideas throughout teams, branches, or the entire company.
  Advantages:
  - Accessible for all interested employees to attend.
  - Potential for interactivity where attendees can ask questions specific to issues they are having.
  - It can be recorded and reused.
  Disadvantages:
  - Planning, finding the right speakers, and settling on a topic is time-consuming
  - Requires organization
  - External experts can cost a lot
  - Requires time to find answer.

HEALTH INFORMATICS STANDARDS

Standards are clear declarations of the level of performance that is anticipated for a healthcare activity. It consists of steps, clinical practise recommendations, treatment protocols, critical paths, algorithms, and declarations of anticipated healthcare results. Health informatics standards establish the requirements for producing high-quality services and confirm how a certain healthcare activity will be carried out in order to achieve the desired results.

Structured terms offer a way to categorize data and establish the semantics of data through standardized, calculable processes. Therefore, health information professionals need the capabilities to concentrate on distributing terminology to software suppliers and organizations in a consistent, high-quality manner via a standard delivery mechanism.

Systematized Nomenclature of Medicine—Clinical Terms (SNOMED CT)

Systematized Nomenclature of Medicine, or SNOMED CT medical professionals and other healthcare professionals use clinical terminology, a defined, multilingual vocabulary of clinical terms, for the electronic transmission of clinical health information.

SNOMED CT currently contains more than 300,000 medical concepts, organized into hierarchies as varied as body structure, clinical findings, geography, and pharmaceutical/biological product, according to the international health terminology standards development organization (IHTSDO), which disseminates the standard. A complex state can be described using multiple concepts at once, each of which is represented by a unique number.

SNOMED CT provides a standard by which medical conditions and symptoms can be referred to, removing any ambiguity that may arise from the use of local or colloquial words. SNOMED CT does this by utilizing numbers to describe medical ideas. The numerical reference system also makes it easier for different healthcare providers and electronic medical record (EMR) systems to interchange clinical data.

Applications of SNOMED CT

- SNOMED CT stands for coded terms that can be utilized in electronic health records to gather, store, and distribute clinical data for use by healthcare organizations.
- SNOMED CT is a crucial component of systems that make it possible to retrieve useful clinical data.
- In the globe, SNOMED CT is the most complete, multilingual clinical healthcare terminology.
- SNOMED CT is a source containing thorough, clinical content that has been verified by science.
- SNOMED CT allows for uniform clinical content representation in electronic health records.
- SNOMED CT is mapped to additional global norms.
- SNOMED CT makes it possible to consistently collect clinical data.
- Support systems can review the record and offer real-time guidance thanks to SNOMED CT.
- SNOMED CT encourages the exchange of pertinent information with other healthcare professionals, enabling all clinicians to understand the information in a similar manner.
- SNOMED CT enables precise and thorough analysis that identifies patients who need follow-up or treatment modifications.
- SNOMED CT breaks down linguistic barriers by allowing multilingual use.
- SNOMED CT facilitates connections between improved clinical guidelines and practises and clinical records.
- SNOMED CT improves the standard of care that patients receive.
- SNOMED CT limits the incidence and effects of unfavorable healthcare occurrences by lowering the expense of unnecessary and redundant testing and treatment.
- SNOMED CT improves the population's access to high-quality, cost-effective care.

Clinical Knowledge and Decision Making

Example of SNOMED CT

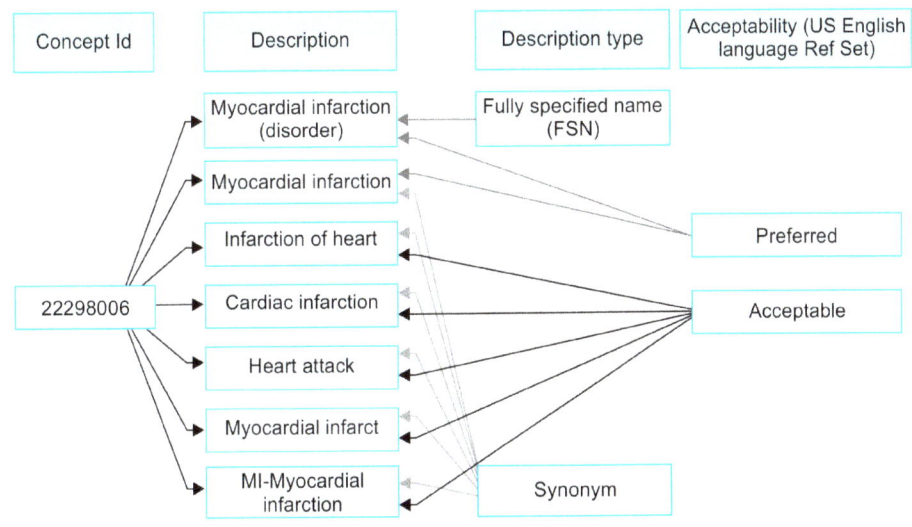

Fig. 6.2: Concept model of SNOMED CT.

SUMMARY

The term "knowledge management" (KM) refers to a collection of organized, methodical steps that an organization can take to get the most out of the knowledge at its disposal. Utilizing the appropriate organizational, social, and managerial initiatives as well as the right technology is typically necessary for effective knowledge management. Gathering, organizing, storing, and disseminating the knowledge required to help the organization expand and thrive is the goal of knowledge management (KM). Utilizing and recycling existing organizational knowledge resources is the main goal of knowledge management (KM), which encourages individuals to look for best practises rather than inventing new ones. Tactic and explicit knowledge are the two forms that knowledge management deals with. It is supported that knowledge is valuable to an organization.

REVIEW QUESTION

1. Define knowledge management system.
2. What is the dimensions of knowledge management system?
3. What are the components of knowledge management system? Explain any two.
4. What are the advantages and challenges of knowledge management system?
5. What are the importance of knowledge management in healthcare and clinical?
6. What is systematized nomenclature of medicine? Give any two examples.
7. What is the applications of SNOMED CT?

MULTIPLE CHOICE QUESTIONS

1. **Knowledge management is:**
   a. A discipline
   b. Based on information
   c. Digital networks as used in an organization
   d. The process of capturing and using expertise
   e. The same as the information value chain

Clinical Knowledge and Decision Making

2. **Tacit knowledge includes expertise that is:**
   a. On paper
   b. In documents
   c. In databases
   d. In people's heads
   e. In e-mail

3. **The KM life cycle includes knowledge:**
   a. Creation
   b. Capture
   c. Organization
   d. Refinement
   e. All of the above are valid

4. **Companies that fail to imbed a viable KM operations probably do not suffer from:**
   a. Building a huge database that is supposed to cater to the entire company
   b. Placing too much emphasis on technology
   c. Having poor leadership
   d. Shortening of the learning curve
   e. Viewing km as a technology or a human resources area

5. **The acceptance of KM has been hindered by:**
   a. The rapid speed of change during the previous ten years
   b. The geographic and worldwide dispersion that has altered the scope of organizations
   c. Lack of knowledge of what Km is and how it helps a business
   d. The attrition and knowledge loss caused by the reengineering and downsizing
   e. Enhanced networking and data communications capabilities

6. **The four-process view of KM includes, in order of sequence:**
   a. Capturing, organizing, refining, and transfer
   b. Organizing, transfer, capturing, and refining
   c. Capturing, refining, organizing, and transfer
   d. Capturing, transfer, refining, and organizing
   e. Capturing, refining, transfer, organizing

7. **In-house development of a KM system is usually:**
   a. Inexpensive
   b. Quick
   c. Highly personalized because they can create it exactly how the business wants it
   d. Answers a and b are accurate
   e. Answers b and c are accurate

8. **The _____ layer of the KM system creates a competitive edge for the learning organization.**
   a. Knowledge-enabling application
   b. Middleware
   c. Transport
   d. Collaborative intelligence and filtering
   e. Authorized access

9. **The least technical of these KM system layers is:**
   a. Physical
   b. Transport
   c. Authorized access control
   d. Middleware
   e. User interface

Answer Key

1. d
2. d
3. e
4. d
5. c
6. a
7. c
8. a
9. e

CHAPTER 7

E-Health: Patient and Internet

At the end of this chapter, student will able to learn about:
- E-health system
- Drivers of e-health
- Use of information and communication technology to improve healthcare (e-health applications)
- Challenges in adopting e-health
- Public health informatics
- Applications of public health informatics
- Role of nurse in public informatics
- The role of public health informatics in enhancing public health

TERMINOLOGIES

- **E-health:** The application of information and communication technology to disciplines linked to and supporting health.
- **M-health:** Using wireless mobile devices for health.
- **Digital health:** It is a broad word that includes e-Health (which also includes m-Health) as well as newer fields like the application of "big data," genomics, and artificial intelligence.
- **Tele-health:** The practice of providing healthcare outside of conventional healthcare facilities using telecommunications and virtual technology.
- **Public health informatics:** The systematic application of information, computer science, and technology to public health practice, research, and education is known as public health informatics.
- **Telemedicine:** Telemedicine takes into account the usage of medical data, also known as Medical Health Records and Electronic Health Records, shared through electronic data exchange.
- **Tele-monitoring:** Use of remote computer processing of patient data (ICD, pacemaker, ECG, blood pressure, glucose levels, etc.) to regularly check on patients' vital signs and symptoms at home.

INTRODUCTION

Health care is a field rich in information and understanding on issues, such as diet, cleanliness, illness prevention, management, and medication-assisted treatment, as well as lifestyle changes. The individual, the doctor, and the community—also known as the pivots of a healthcare system—all own this continuously generated knowledge. In order to provide high-quality healthcare to a larger population, providers must build and run more cost-effective facilities, lower operating expenses, boost productivity, and increase efficiency by effectively managing patient flows and making the best use of expensive technology and labor.

Healthcare professionals now have the tools they need to identify and treat a wider range of issues and illnesses because to technological advancements. They can be used to identify and cure illnesses, stop disease from spreading, keep patients healthy, or make health services more accessible. The integration and coordination of healthcare might lead to the best possible utilization of expensive and scarce resources. Networked health systems and patients have access to seamless, coordinated, and ongoing treatment through utilizing information and communication technologies to deliver improved healthcare services in disadvantaged areas. With the development of modern telecommunications, information processing power, and health diagnostic equipment downsizing, it is now possible to provide more immediate and efficient healthcare to the general public.

E-HEALTH SYSTEM

Definition

The World Health Organization (WHO) defines e-Health as "the application of information and communication technologies to support health and health-related sectors." The use of telecommunications and digital technology, such as computers, the Internet, and mobile devices, to support health services and health improvement.

Drivers of E-Health

Applications of electronic communications in the healthcare sector can be very advantageous. Information, a range of functions that need extensive communication and a variety of stakeholders define healthcare services. The benefits of e-universal health's reach, speed, and seamless connectivity can improve the provision of healthcare through public health upkeep, education of healthcare professionals, facilitation of collaboration among health sciences researchers, enhancement of access to high-quality care, and cost reduction through process simplification. The future of telemedicine and e-health technology may be altered by patients' desire for online communication with their medical professionals. Current e-health growth is mostly fueled by:

Consumer Inclinations

- A growing percentage of people are utilizing online resources for health-related information.
- The need for more involvement and participation in controlling one's health status.
- The need for diversified services, individualized care, and equal access.
- The requirement for quick access to specialized information and experience.
- The ease of reporting health metrics.

Technological Aptitudes
- Using electronic communications to increase accessibility, connectivity, and speed.
- The ability of electronic communications to transcend limitations of geography, time, and location.
- Benefits of electronic communication in the highly information- and communication-intensive profession of healthcare.
- The accessibility of portable, network-enabled medical diagnostic and monitoring devices.

Health System Policy
- To improve current skills, widen the audience, and make the best use of limited resources.
- Using integrated delivery networks (IDNs), to supply entire health services (care, content, commerce, convenience, and connection).

USE OF INFORMATION AND COMMUNICATION TECHNOLOGY TO IMPROVE HEALTHCARE (E-HEALTH APPLICATIONS)

The great potential for numerous applications that will change the way we work, study, and live has been brought about by the communication age. One industry in particular that is undergoing an intriguing shift as a result of the integration of these telecommunications technologies is healthcare. The healthcare sector is rapidly recognizing IT as a key resource for delivering on-demand health-related information services and decision support, managing changing organizational needs and rising expenses, enhancing the caliber of patient care, preventing sickness, and promoting wellness. Virtually all diseases and conditions have online support groups, and there are a virtually endless number of conversation topics for each disease category. The internet is widely employed in medical education as a delivery method for online learning programmes as well as a learning tool to supplement formal curricula. When students are geographically spread out, web-based learning can be helpful to assist clinical education. For instance, clinical skills can be learned through video demonstrations. The following categories can be used to classify e-health applications:

Consumer Health
- Online resources for consumer health.
- Electronic medical records (EMRs) for access to comprehensive patient health information. Internet-based communication between patients, physicians, and providers.
- Home care for elderly individuals and others with chronic illnesses to manage their health.

Clinical Care
- Telemedicine using remote diagnosis, monitoring, and treatment.
- Clinical transactions, such as bookkeeping, billing, purchasing, inventory management, and reporting of test results.
- Clinical decision assistance in the form of guidelines for diagnosis, warnings about potential drug interactions, allergy triggers, or any other clinical event needing rapid care, and prompts to follow up on standard procedures.

Administrative and Financial Transactions
- Service payments made electronically.
- Management of claims online.
- The administrative exchange of health information via electronic means between providers.

Public Health
- Monitoring community health
- Integrating healthcare resources for better decision-making
- Managing disasters

Professional Training
- Continuing medical education for rural medical workers
- Online training and education for health professionals
- Conference webcasting and grand rounds television broadcast
- Surgical training simulations

Clinical Research
- Internet-based databases for biomedicine
- Remote control of research equipment
- Electronic research data dissemination is a convenient, affordable

According to WHO, E-Health is the secure and cost-effective application of information and communication technologies (ICT) to the advancement of health and sectors associated with it. It includes a variety of interventions, such as wearable technology, big data, tele-health, telemedicine, mobile health (m-Health), and even artificial intelligence. Universal health coverage (UHC) and the sustainable development goals are two major health targets that have been acknowledged as being crucially dependent on e-Health (SDGs).

- Enhancing and expanding the application of ICT in the advancement of health.
- Establishing standards and frameworks for evaluation to assist in the selection, adoption, management, and evaluation of e-health solutions by Member States in order to promote sound investment and governance.
- By using a coordinated multi-stakeholder and multi-sectoral approach, Member States will get technical help and guidance as they integrate e-health solutions into their national e-health agendas.
- To guide national policy and practice, as well as to periodically report on the usage of e-Health in the region, monitoring and reporting on advances and trends in digital innovation for public health is necessary.
- Fostering cross-organizational cooperation and coordination with a view to enhancing coordinated methods for putting into practice and expanding cost-effective e-Health solutions.

CHALLENGES IN ADOPTING E-HEALTH

Even while e-health has many exciting advantages, there are still a number of barriers preventing consumers and health organizations from adopting it widely. The majority of customers are still unaware that they can acquire specialized information online. A number of legal issues are raised by the use of electronic communication in medicine, including the doctor's responsibility of confidentiality, the patient's right to informed consent, the elements of a medical record, accepted usage and practise guidelines, state licensure, and product endorsement. Physicians are unlikely to accept clinical information systems when they conflict with established practise practices. Before it can be fully included into the system of healthcare as a whole, e-health must first overcome a number of obstacles.

These can be:
- System design and reliability restrictions.
- Appropriate infrastructure is required.
- Networks must have a compatible hardware and software environment.
- Adjusting user needs to different degrees of knowledge among medical professionals.
- Insufficient end-user training.
- Inadequate sharing of knowledge and the distribution of evaluation results.
- Lack of knowledge regarding the existence of internet health resources.
- Discovering reliable, pertinent information online can be challenging.
- Need to appease a variety of stakeholders with competing agendas, needs, and expectations.
- Under circumstances of erratic demand, there is a requirement for prompt service response.
- Reluctance to depart from customary methods.
- Services must be integrated into the administrative, technical, and medical staff's workflow.
- Lack of clear guidelines for preserving the confidentiality and privacy of medical records.
- Issues relating to medical malpractice liability, medical professional credentialing, and interstate licensure.
- Lack of appropriate payment methods.
- Linguistic diversity, cultural diversity, and variations in medical practice.
- Lack of touch as a means of communication.
- Lack of formality and relative anonymity.
- There is no explicit protocol on how to pay for electronic consultations.
- Lack of long-term financing strategies.
- Maintaining cost management while keeping up with the rapidly evolving technology.

PUBLIC HEALTH INFORMATICS

Informatics is still in the early phases of transforming public health. To date, informatics in public health has largely been relegated to "pushing the broom" at the end of the parade rather than recognizing the full potential benefits that would accrue from their involvement at the outset, public health has tended to bring in informaticists to help resolve systemic issues like non-interoperability. Public health informatics differs from other informatics specialty areas in a number of ways, albeit sharing many similarities with them. These include a focus on information science and technology applications that improve population health rather than individual health, a focus on disease prevention rather than treatment, a focus on preventive intervention at all vulnerable points in the causal chains leading to disease, injury, or disability, and operation within an institutional rather than a personal context.

Definition

The systematic application of information, computer science, and technology to public health practice, research, and education is known as public health informatics.

Application

- To spot and address issues with community health, keep track of health status.
- Determine and research the community's health issues and dangers.
- People should be informed, educated, and empowered about health issues.
- Encourage community involvement and action to find solutions to health issues.
- Create plans and policies to aid in promoting the health of the person and the community.
- Enforce laws and rules that promote safety and health.
- Ensure the provision of healthcare when otherwise unavailable and connect them to the necessary personal health services.
- Ensure a skilled workforce in both public and private healthcare.
- Analyze the efficiency, usability, and excellence of individual and community-based health services.
- Research into fresh perspectives and creative answers to health issues.
- Gathering and keeping records of life-changing events like births and deaths.
- Infectious illness surveillance involves gathering information on reported cases of communicable diseases from physicians, hospitals, and labs.
- Exchanging data and trends on infectious diseases with other groups, including the general public.
- Gathering data on lead screening and vaccination of children.
- Gathering and studying data from emergency rooms to find early signs of biological dangers.
- Gathering information on hospital capacity to enable emergency response planning.

Role of Nurse

Nurse's responsibility in public informatics is to advance public health. In this role, nurses concentrate on facilitating access to care for those who are underserved and at risk. Through evidence-based care and education, public health nurses work to lower health risks and assist prevent disease at the population level. The responsibilities of public health nurses include:
- Collecting and studying general medical data
- Assessing individuals' health and developing treatment regimens
- Keeping an eye on patients' conditions for any changes
- Providing high-quality care with doctors
- Providing information to patients about available resources and assisting them in receiving care
- Putting a focus on primary prevention to stop illness or harm before it happens
- Collaborating with public health professionals to increase access to care for marginalized communities
- Establishing a rapport with patients and monitoring their development
- Directing patients to different specialists as necessary

- Analyzing local community health patterns
- Managing public health programme budgets

The Role of Public Health Informatics in Enhancing Public Health

- **Planning and system design:** It involve determining which data and sources are most effective for achieving a surveillance goal, as well as who will have access to it, how they will do so, and under what circumstances. They also involve enhancing analysis and action by enhancing the interaction of the surveillance system with other information systems.
- **Data collection:** It includes identifying potential biases associated with various data collection techniques, (such as telephone use or cultural attitudes toward technology), determining the most appropriate use of structured data in comparison to free text, the most helpful vocabulary, and data standards, and recommending technologies (such as global positioning systems and radio-frequency identification) to support simpler, quicker, and higher-quality data entry in the field.
- **Interpretation:** Understanding the value of comparing data from various surveillance programmes (connected by time, place, person, or condition) in order to gain new views and combining data from various sources and of varying quality in order to provide an interpreting context.
- **Dissemination:** It includes recognizing advantages for data producers, recommending the best ways to reach the target audience, and recommending appropriate information displays for consumers.
- **Application to public health programmes:** Evaluating the value of having surveillance data flow directly into information systems that support public health interventions, as well as information components or standards that facilitate this linkage of surveillance to action, and improving access to and use of information produced by a surveillance system for field personnel and healthcare professionals.

SUMMARY

ICTs (information and communications technologies) have the potential to significantly improve both individual and community healthcare. ICTs can assist in bridging the information gaps that have developed in the health sector of developing and new industrial countries—between healthcare professionals and the communities they serve as well as between the authors of health research and the practitioners who require it—by offering new and more effective ways of accessing, communicating, and storing information. ICTs can also increase the effectiveness of the health system and reduce medical errors through the creation of databases and other applications. It is a difficult undertaking to make sure that e-health develops into a good, commonplace medium for providing medical services. E-health must ensure that clinical care transactions take place predictably, efficiently, and without jeopardising patient safety. It must also connect the players in these transactions. E-capacity health's to "flatten" organizational hierarchies, facilitate dynamic information flows between enterprises, and empower consumers may need the development of new operational strategies, economic models, service delivery models, and management methods. While reducing the risks connected with e-health service delivery, organizations must assess the possibilities and implications of e-health, anticipate healthcare demands, and are ready to adapt to local conditions.

REVIEW QUESTION

1. Define public informatics.
2. Explain the applications of public informatics.
3. Explain the challenges in implementing public informatics in India.
4. Explain the role of nurse in public informatics.
5. Define E-health and its application in nursing.
6. Explain the use of information and communication technology to improve healthcare.

MULTIPLE CHOICE QUESTIONS

1. **Electronic health record can be accessed by _____ whereas electronic medical records can be accessed by _____.**
   a. Multiple facilities; a single facility
   b. A single facility; multiple facilities
   c. Patients; doctors
   d. Doctors; patients

2. **New model of Health Information Management (HIM) practice is _____.**
   a. Terminology focused
   b. Information focused
   c. Disease focused
   d. Condition focused

3. **HIT stands for:**
   a. Health information tables
   b. Health information transcription
   c. Health information technology
   d. Health information terminology

4. **What is a comprehensive technology system that allows hospitals to manage all aspects of operation:**
   a. Health information system
   b. Hospital information system
   c. Hospital management model
   d. Health management model

5. **Filing, indexing and retrieving records is work carried in:**
   a. Therapeutic
   b. Medical records department
   c. Administration department
   d. Maintenance department

Answer Key

1. c   2. c   3. c   4. a   5. b

CHAPTER 8

Using Information in Healthcare Management

At the end of this chapter, student will able to learn about:
- Nursing informatics
- Types of nursing information system
- Purposes of nursing information system
- Components of nursing information system
- Importance of evaluation, analysis and presentation of healthcare data
- Healthcare data in decision making

TERMINOLOGIES

- **Nursing information**: It includes data collected by nurses, data used by nurses, data regarding nursing activities, and data about the nursing resource are all examples of nursing information.
- **Information system:** An information system is a collection of interconnected sets of components that work together to gather, store, and process data as well as deliver information.
- **Nursing information system:** To organize and transform data into knowledge for use in nursing practice, a nursing information system combines nursing, information science, and computer science.
- **Healthcare data:** Information gathered from medical test results, hospital records, investigation findings, and other data sources.
- **Data analytics:** The science of analyzing raw data to draw inferences and interpretations regarding information gathered through various information systems is known as data analytics.
- **Clinical decision:** Clinical decision making is a continuous, evolving process that uses data analysis to choose evidence-based courses of action for improved health outcomes.

NURSING INFORMATION SYSTEMS

Introduction

The acquisition and implementation of nursing information systems in the acute sector have received recent attention. The resource management programme gave hospitals the chance to think about the best ways to assist nursing with information and information technology (IT). It was necessary for nurses to express their information needs rapidly. Numerous choices must be made while selecting a computer system, and the speed of progress unavoidably brought up its own issues.

Nursing informatics is a specialty within the nursing sector that processes patient data and aids in medical decision-making by fusing nursing science and information technology. Computers and portable devices are used by computer nurses to manage massive volumes of electronic medical records. These specialized nurses assess the usability of their computer systems as well to ensure swift and accurate data retrieval. Finding patient information in one electronic format, modifying it, and putting it into another are some crucial elements of this discipline. Applying nursing principles to electronic data in order to offer the best possible care for patients is another daily task in the field of nursing computers.

Definition

Nursing information systems (NIS) are computerized programmes that organize and handle clinical data from a range of healthcare settings in order to help nurses provide better patient care.

A database and at least one nursing classification language, such as North American Nursing Diagnosis Association (NANDA), Nursing Intervention Classification (NIC), and Nursing Diagnosis Extension and Classification, are used in the design of the majority of Nursing information systems in order to accomplish this (NDEC).

Purposes of Nursing Informatics System

- To improve communication within the team
- To supply a system for collecting data
- To ease the burden of paperwork and quality control paper loss
- Describe nursing interventions and their results
- To compile knowledge that a doctor might not be able to recall.

Nursing Information System Components

The use of nursing processes and activities is supported by nursing information systems, which also offer tools for managing the provision of nursing care. Consequently, different NIS components include the following:

A System for Managing and Documenting Nursing Care

Similar functionalities are provided by the medical documentation system and the nurse management and documentation system. The so-called nursing process, which primarily consists of nursing patient history, nursing care planning with problem definition, formulation of nursing goals, and planning of nursing tasks, then execution of nursing tasks, and evaluation of results, must be supported by the nursing management and documentation system. The nursing management and documentation system supports the use of nursing classifications and terminologies such NANDA, NIC, and NOC **(Fig. 8.1)**.

Using Information in Healthcare Management

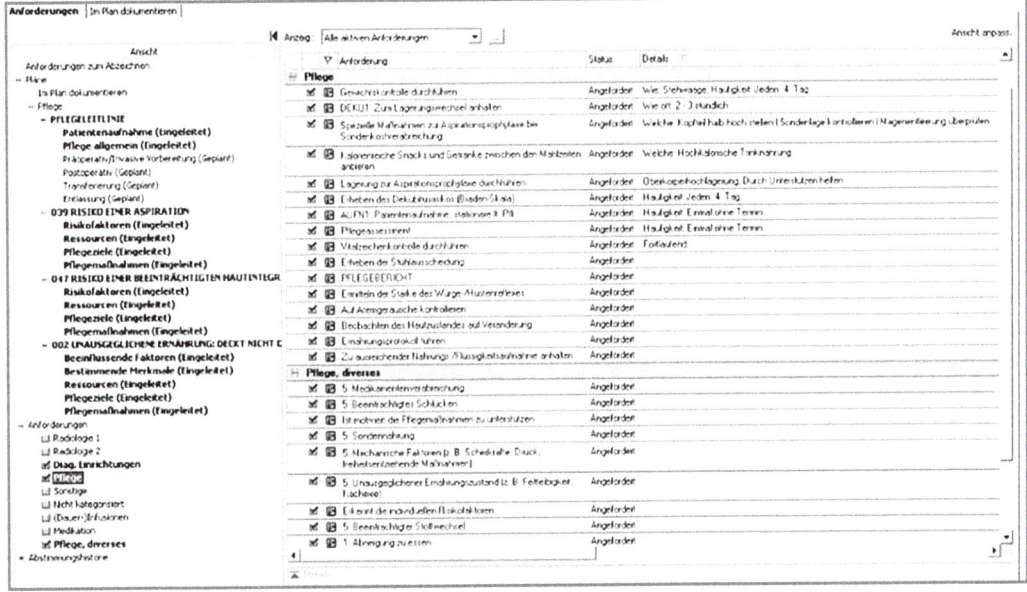

Fig. 8.1: Documenting nursing care.

Nursing Procedures and Records

The delivery of patient care revolves around the nursing process. Throughout the nursing process continuum, data and information are constantly presented to nurses. Each step of the nursing process incorporates data and information:
- Assessment
- Diagnosis
- Planning
- Implementation
- Evaluation

Information management depends heavily on nursing documentation, which is sometimes seen as the sixth step in the nursing process. In order to identify the desired outcome, nurses must document completely and accurately.
- Work lists to remind staff of scheduled nursing actions
- Clinical information systems and point-of-care systems
- Computer-generated client documentation
- Monitoring tools that enter vital signs and other measurements directly into the patient record (CPR) and electronic medical record (EMR)
- Critical pathways, automatic invoicing for supplies or procedures, and nursing documentation created by computers

The System of Clinical and Essential Routes

Clinical pathways for patient-centered treatments are taught to healthcare professionals using established knowledge bases that include data on family history, allergies, drug reactions, clinical activity sequences, and evidence-based medical history. With assistance from CIS and HIS, they also carry out the actual treatment based on customized clinical pathways under the supervision of the knowledge service application platform **(Fig. 8.2)**.

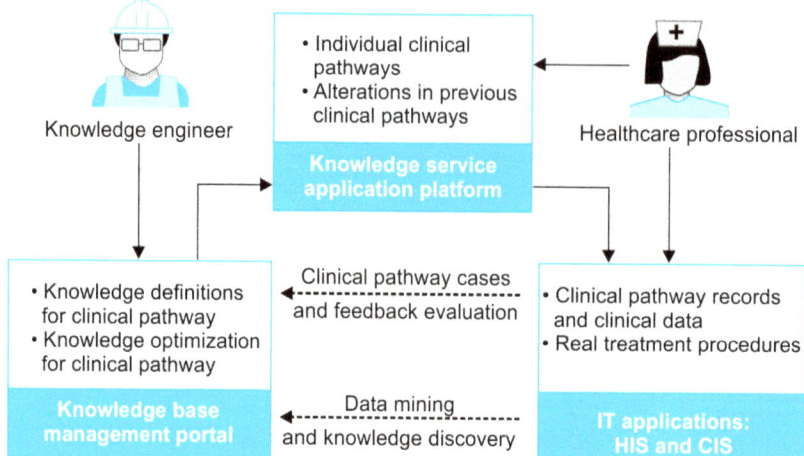

Fig. 8.2: Clinical pathway model.

The linked knowledge may be mined from the stored cases in the CIS and HIS to further enhance the therapy because clinical pathway systems are evidence-based knowledge tools that govern the treatment through collaboration among several medical care sections. Clinical pathway systems can help medical practitioners assess and analyze treatment deviations for various patients in order to prevent recurring mistakes or variations in the future. This reduces the cost of treatment while ultimately improving medical services.

Patient Record System

The system allows for the structured or free text entry of a patient's vital signs, admission and nursing assessments, care plan, and nursing notes. When required, these can be obtained from a centralized repository **(Figs. 8.3 and 8.4)**.

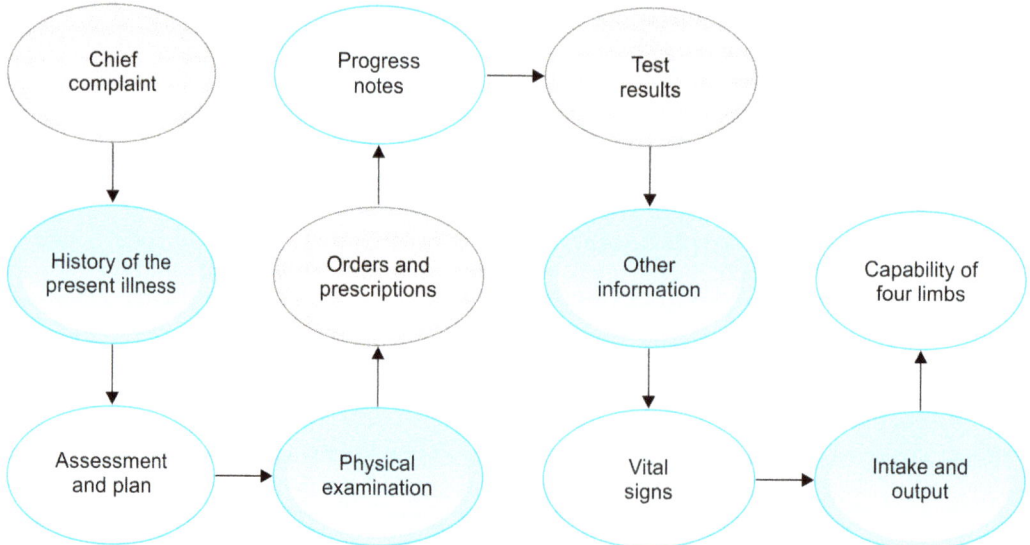

Fig. 8.3: Patient record system.

Using Information in Healthcare Management

- Data = 9:00 am −100mg/dL, 4:00 pm 180 mg/dL
- Information =

Time	Glucose
9.00 am	100 mg/dL
4.00 pm	180 mg/dL

- Knowledge = My clients glucose level rises in the late afternoon. His insulin dose needs to be adjusted

Fig. 8.4: Progress report in patient record system.

STAFF DUTY CHART

Staff Name	Date January	1	2	3	4	5	6	7
Staff 1	Plan							
	Actual							
Staff 2	Plan							
	Actual							
Staff 2	Plan							
	Actual							
Staff 4	Plan							
	Actual							
Staff 5	Plan							
	Actual							
Staff 6	Plan							
	Actual							
Staff 7	Plan							
	Actual							
Sfaff 8	Plan							
	Actual							

Legend	
07:00 - 15:00	M
15:00 - 23:00	A
23:00 - 06:00	N
Weekly off	WO

Fig. 8.5: Nursing duty schedule.

Nursing Staff Administration

Using the scheduling guidelines supplied in the shift modules, nurses can self-plan their shifts. An administrator or manager who is in charge of scheduling can subsequently confirm or modify the shifts. Shift modules are made to deal with staffing numbers, overtime, absences, and cost-effective staffing **(Fig. 8.5)**.

Clinical Data Integration

Nursing staff can retrieve, view, and analyze clinical data from all disciplines here before integrating it into a patient's care plan. Clinical pathway support system is involved **(Fig. 8.6)**.

Fig. 8.6: Case management through clinical data integration.

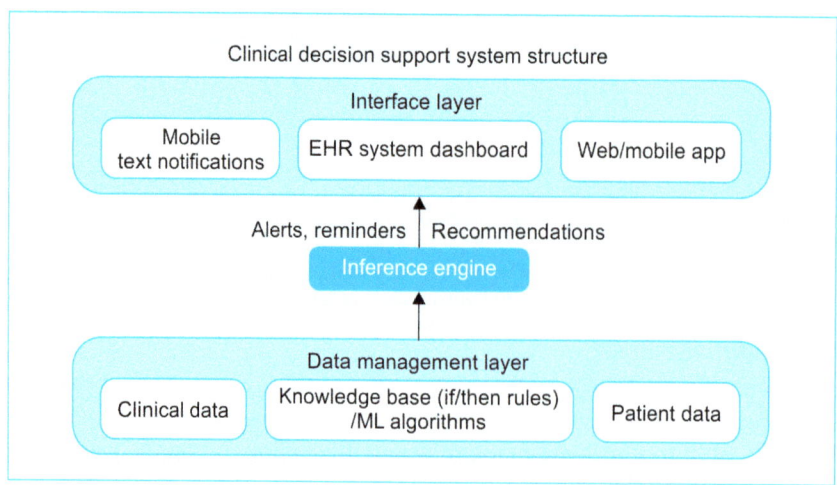

Fig. 8.7: Decision support system.

Using Information in Healthcare Management

Decision Support System

Decision support modules can be added to nursing information systems, and they offer prompts and reminders as well as maps out the relationships between illness etiologies/related factors, signs/symptoms, and patient populations. Medical resources can also be made accessible online **(Fig. 8.7)**.

System for Case Management

Case management is the most current advancement in the way that nursing care is delivered. It represents a return to nursing practises that were common before hospitals were the primary setting for patient care in many ways. Using communication and the resources at hand, case management is a collaborative process that analyzes, plans, implements, coordinates, monitors, and evaluates options and services to suit an individual's requirements and promotes high-quality, cost-effective results. Case management nursing models have changed throughout time. These are distinguished by either a "external" focus in which the case manager supervises clients and the provision of services across the continuum of an organization, or a "internal" focus in which the case manager works within a treatment facility **(Fig. 8.8)**.

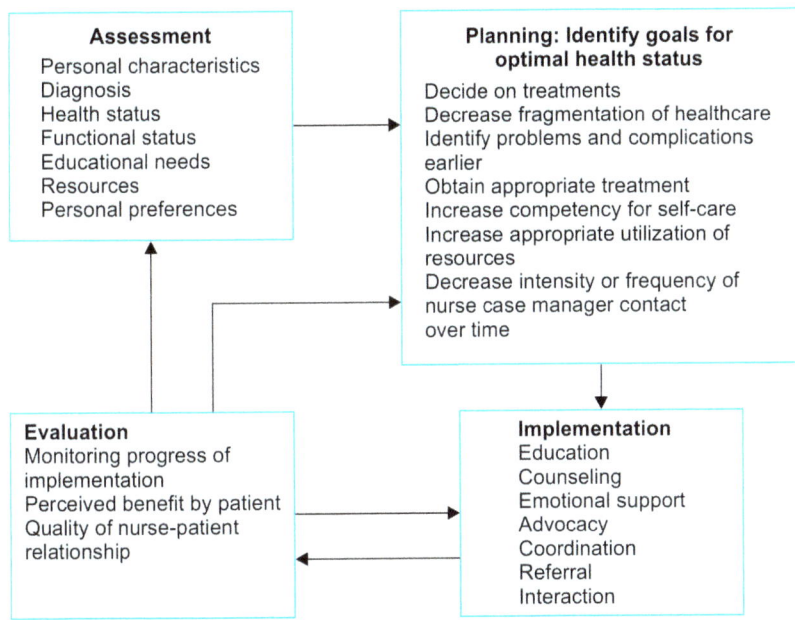

Fig. 8.8: Example of case management model.

System for Nursing Activity

Excretion, decubitus, hair and nail care, skin care, wound treatment, body cleaning, oral and dental care, nutrition and liquid balance, and thrombosis are among the nursing treatments that are carried out as scheduled. Documentation is required for each patient care procedure, as well as for any changes to the care plan or effects on the patient's health status. Facts pertaining to therapy must be disclosed to the accountable doctor **(Fig. 8.9)**.

Using Information in Healthcare Management

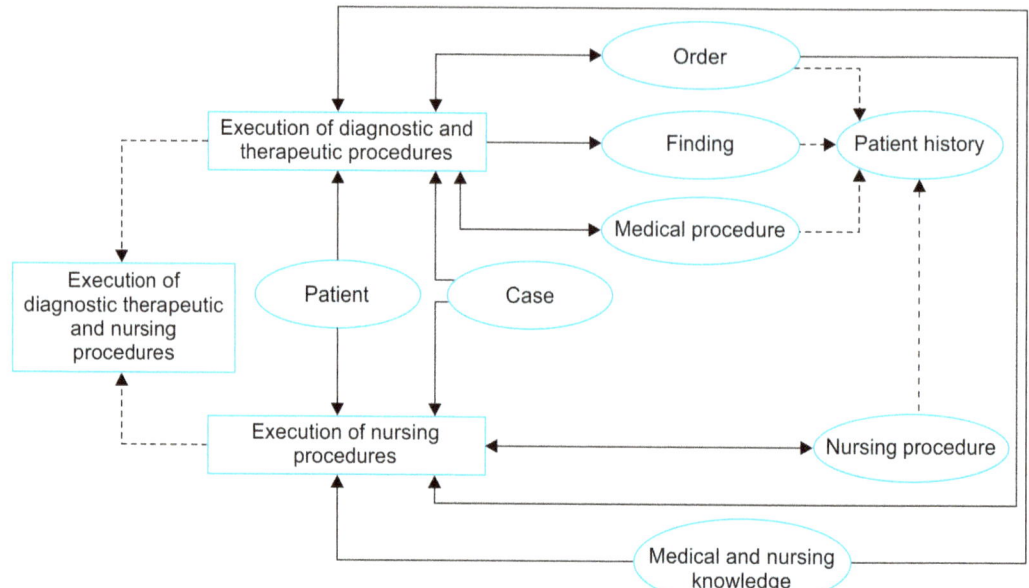

Fig. 8.9: Nursing activity pathway.

Nursing Discharge and Medical Report Writing (Fig. 8.10)

Nursing discharge entails completing of documentation and writing of a nursing report by the attending nurse. The nursing report comprises, for example:
- Information about activity level
- Diet, and wound care

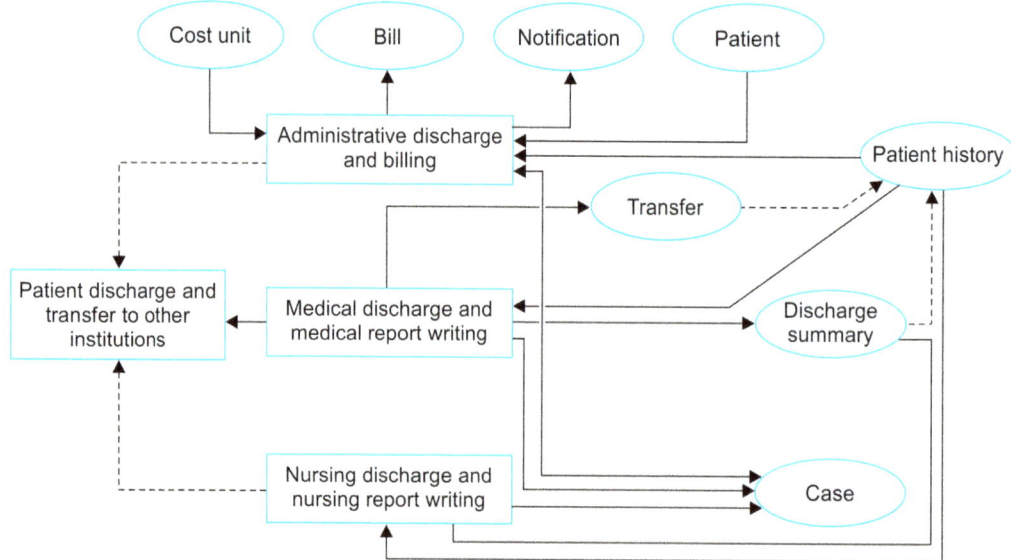

Fig. 8.10: Patient discharge and transfer to other institutions.

Classification Method for Patients

PCSs offer precise clinical data for forecasting and resource allocation. A PCS provides the data required for processes like budgeting, accounting, and managing human resources, among other management duties. Additionally, it evaluates and categorizes patients based on the severity of their illness, the need for care, and the nursing activities required to meet those needs for a certain time frame **(Fig. 8.11)**.

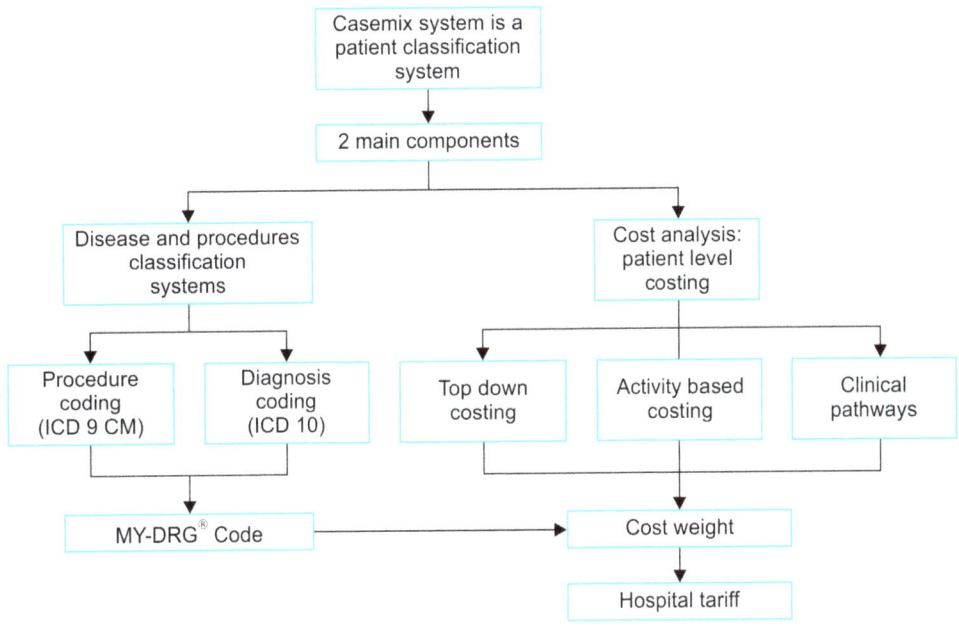

Fig. 8.11: Casemix evidence based system model of patient classification.

Nursing Information Systems Provide Several Benefits (Fig. 8.12)

- **Better workload functionality:** The shift modules make it easier to decide on staffing numbers and the right balance of skills for each shift. Roster design and revision take less time as a result.
- **Better care planning:** Less time is spent on care planning, and the information that is captured is of higher quality. As a result, care planning, assessments, and evaluations are more thorough.
- **Improved medication administration:** Because electronic prescriptions are easier to read, it is less likely that patients may receive the erroneous medication.

Nursing Informatics and Technological Skill Requirements

- Improve patient education, increase accessibility of care, and document and assess patient care using information and communication technologies.
- To evaluate and keep track of patients, use the proper technologies.
- Assemble a multidisciplinary team to decide how to use technology and gather data in an ethical manner.

Using Information in Healthcare Management

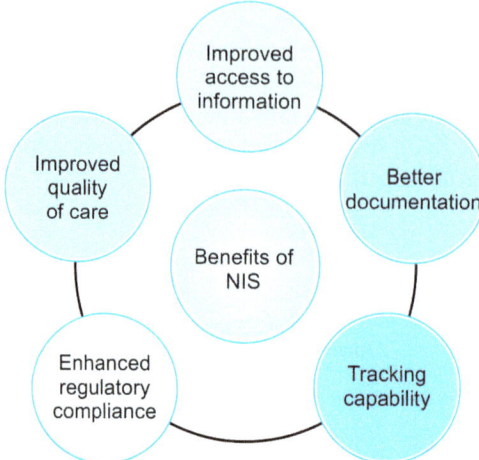

Fig. 8.12: Benefits of nursing information system.

- Modify technology utilization to accommodate patient demands.
- Inform patients about medical technology.
- Maintain patient confidentiality and safety when using information technology in healthcare.
- Make better use of information technologies to expand one's understanding.

Future Developments in Nursing Information Technology

Information technology advancements highlighted the necessity for all nurses to:
- Include data from assessing patients' healthcare requirements.
- Develop care plans.
- Providing other medical providers with patient information.
- In fact, nurses work in an atmosphere that is information-intensive.
- Acquire better knowledge of health information concepts and the technology used to organize and analyze information.
- Nursing practise methods will change to take use of automation as technology develops more.
- Nursing practitioners will move around a lot and play important roles in incorporating technology into patient care.
- Because they collect and document data, have a global perspective on systems, set priorities, oversee all aspects of care, and comprehend the necessity for patient information access, nurses make good information systems professionals.
- Despite the advantages nursing information systems provide, they are not frequently employed in healthcare and, where they have been implemented, they have not been well-received. This is likely a result of inadequate training and a failure to inform the end-user of the rationale behind its implementation. Furthermore, there hasn't been much research done to assess the financial advantages or cost-effectiveness of these information systems.

EVALUATION, ANALYSIS AND PRESENTATION OF HEALTHCARE DATA TO INFORM DECISIONS

Introduction

Healthcare practitioners constantly struggle to get and extract medical data, in large part because data and technology are not integrated, forcing manual and time-consuming process. This relative lack of data accessibility and integration often results in valuable data going undetected as productivity and workflow needs continue to rise. The information is there, but it is useless because it cannot be accessed. By having healthcare professionals repeat tests and studies that may not have been necessary if the entire complement of medical data had been readily available at the point of service, this has the potential to cause data redundancy. Additionally, when medical professionals make judgments about diagnosis and treatment without having complete and conclusive data, data accessibility issues can negatively impact healthcare results.

Definition

Data Analytics

The healthcare sector produces a lot of data, but it has a hard time turning that data into insights that enhance patient outcomes and operational effectiveness. The goal of data analytics in healthcare is to assist practitioners in overcoming barriers to the widespread use of data-derived intelligence:

- Providing accurate data-driven forecasts in real-time to help healthcare providers respond more swiftly to changing healthcare markets and environments.
- Making healthcare data easier to share among coworkers and external partners, as well as easier to visualise for the general public.
- Increasing data innovation and collaboration amongst healthcare companies to turn analytics-ready data into information that is ready for business by automating low-impact data management chores.

The tools used in analytics fall into three general categories:

1. Data-gathering software that uses patient questionnaires, case files, and machine-to-machine data exchanges as its data sources.
2. Programs that clean, validate, and analyze data in answer to a particular research topic software that builds on the findings of the analysis to suggest various actions to reach particular healthcare objectives.
3. Analytics software must safeguard the data and the analysis results in addition to gathering, analyzing, and interpreting data. It must also make sure that the healthcare professionals who will profit from the insights have ready access to the information in a format that they can utilize in their work.

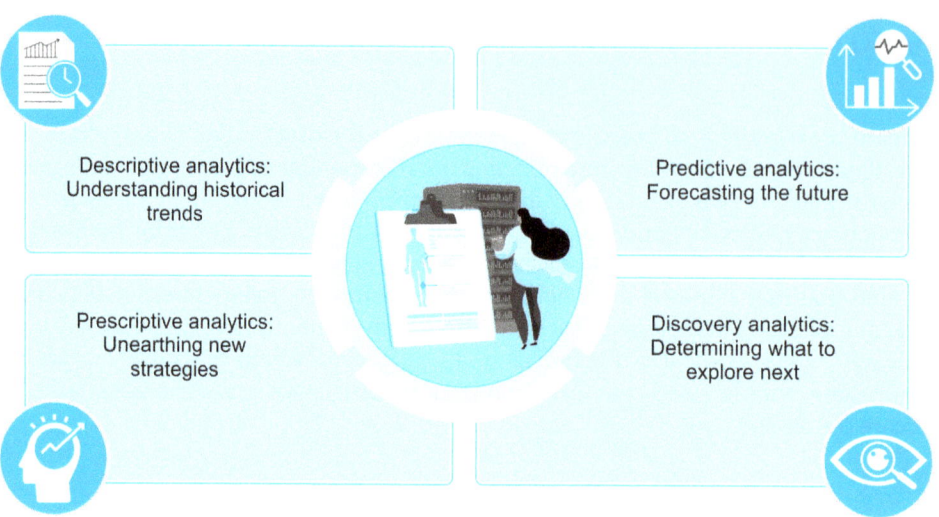

Fig. 8.13: Four types of healthcare data analytics.

TYPES OF DATA ANALYTICS (FIG. 8.13)

Descriptive Analytics

Providers can concentrate on current clinical problems and investigate the causes of increased or decreased outcomes thanks to descriptive analytics. For instance, caregivers could look at how many patients require the pneumococcal vaccine or how many diabetic patients have their blood sugar under control.

Predictive Analytics

Readmissions are the most prevalent problem that healthcare institutions must address under the value-based care model. Providers employ predictive analytics to estimate a potential percentage in order to ensure that the proportion of patients returning to the hospital is as low as possible. Additionally, by considering the health risks, behaviors, lifestyles, pre-existing diseases, and comorbidities of the patient, caregivers can anticipate days of stay and look into potential admissions. This information can be used to predict emergency room use.

Prescriptive Analytics

Prescriptive analytics implies helping caregivers measuring and managing patient population health, like focusing patients with obesity and diabetes and assess their LDL levels or other measurements. *WHO* has multiple tools for prescriptive analytics and population health monitoring, e.g. calculators of child mortality, health disparities, HIV prevalence and more.

Discovery Analytics

Data discovery is the process of navigating or applying advanced analytics to data to detect informative patterns that could not have been discovered otherwise.

DATA MANAGEMENT

The Healthcare Information System (HIS) was created to make it possible to collect, store, and then make information available for both primary and secondary use. Data or information used primarily for operational purposes is referred to as primary usage (i.e. caring for the patient). The term "secondary use" describes the usage of data for tasks like auditing and research that are not directly related to the patient's real care. In both cases, raw or calculated data about a single patient or a group of patients are presented.

Data Source and Database Creation

- **Computerized generated data:** Imaging modalities and information system technologies, such as picture archiving and communication system (PACS), computerized physician order entry (CPOE), and radiology information system (RIS), are the main focus of computerized sources for imaging data. Additionally crucial, manual data entry has historically been a crucial data source in imaging practise.
- **Physician order related data:** The ordering clinician, who in theory is accountable for supplying imaging professionals with pertinent, correct, and thorough clinical data at the time of order entry, is another significant human source of clinical data. The selection of the imaging exam, protocol optimization, interpretation, and reporting are only a few of the imaging chain processes that depend on the quality and volume of this clinical data. Even with the adoption of CPOE systems, order entry clinical data input is very frequently inadequate because they can be "gamed" by entering inaccurate clinical data that is only needed to fulfill order entry requirements.
- **Classification of data**
  - Medical data can be loosely categorized into three classes based on how quickly things change over time. These can be divided into three groups: dynamic, episodic, and static.
  - Genetic information and family history are examples of static data that are very steady over time and require little updating after being added to a database. Episodic data, on the other hand, tends to be pretty consistent through time with the odd episodic change (e.g., medical problem list, surgical history, pharmacology). These episodic changes can act as internal cues for database adjustment because they are frequently linked to significant medical occurrences like hospitalization or a change in healthcare providers. A number of high-yield data sources (such as discharge summaries and billing records) can be used in the case of a patient who, for instance, is hospitalized (resulting in new episodic data).
  - Dynamic data is composed of medical information that is always undergoing change and fresh information. This kind of information is frequently the consequence of new or evolving medical issues, which may necessitate more diagnostic test results (such as laboratory or imaging data), referrals and consultations, or treatment measures (e.g., pharmacologic, surgical). Physician order entry data, consultation reports, progress notes, and laboratory/imaging reports are just a few examples of the data sources that can be used to create dynamic data in an electronic patient record. This data is constantly changing, making it the most challenging to update and guarantee accuracy. One would anticipate improvements in retrieval and recording of dynamic data mining as computerized data mining algorithms and artificial intelligence approaches continue to evolve.

DATA MANAGEMENT PROCESS

Data management is a set of activities consisting of **(Fig. 8.14)**:
- Generating data
- Data gathering (collection, gathering, capture)
- Data exchange
- Data archiving
- Data exploitation
- Data evaluation
- Interpreting data
- Data presentation
- Dissemination of data
- Data acquisition and generation

Instead of providing aggregate data on all patients, health data sources and generation focus on fundamental patient health data relating to each individual's condition. The following categories of health data sources can be made based on individual patients.

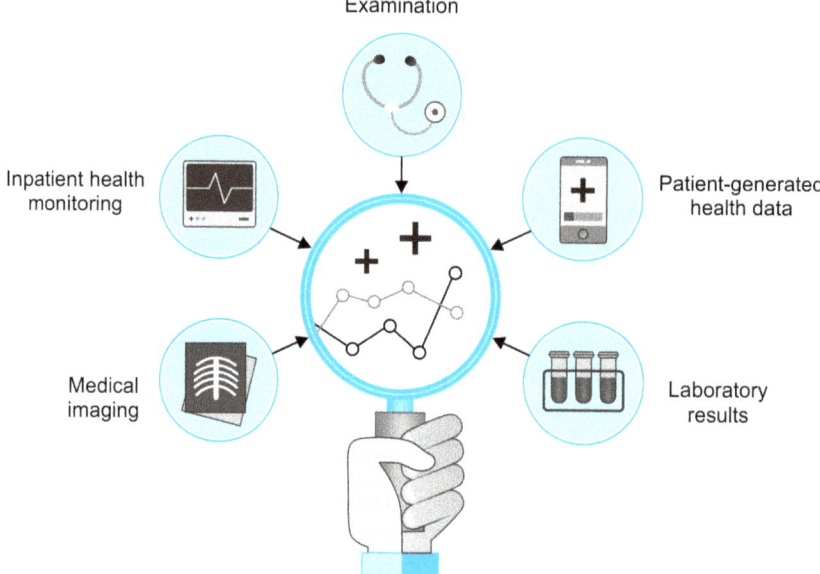

Fig. 8.14: Data generating sources in healthcare.

Examination

When a doctor evaluates a patient's condition (whether during a first visit or a follow-up), the following data is acquired and recorded in the electronic health record:

Using Information in Healthcare Management

Personal data	Health data	Transaction data
• Sex • Age • Occupation • Date of birth • Marital status • Insurance • Contacts and more	• Chief complaint (CC) • Symptoms (frequency in urination, skin rash, stomachache, cough, etc.) • Comorbidities, traumas • Vitals (temperature, pulse rate, respiration rate, blood pressure, and more depending on symptoms) • Lab results (if available, including blood, urine, other body fluids tests) • Lifestyle choices (physical activity, habits, nutrition, etc.) • Diagnosis (primary, secondary) • Treatment (medications, procedures, etc.) • Childhood diseases • Family diseases • Allergies	Claims and other billing records (if available)

Patient-generated Health Data (PGHD)

PGHD refers to the kind of information that the patient or their loved ones supply. Currently, mobile health apps, portable medical devices, and smart wearables are the most common ways to collect and share PGHD. CGMs, smart watches, insulin pumps, activity trackers, oximeters, Holter monitors, handheld capnographs, smart phones, and other devices can all be used by patients to collect data. After that, specific m-Health apps can synchronize this data and send it to a caregiver.

Both subjective and objective PGHD are possible. Weight, heart rate and activity, blood pressure, blood glucose, temperature, oximetry readings, and more are examples of objective data. Subjective refers to the patient's state of mind, sleep, pain, itching, etc.

In order for doctors to have a more complete view of the patient's health status, patient-generated health data is meant to supplement clinical data acquired during appointments, tests, and procedures. PGHD is particularly useful for managing chronic diseases and recovering after surgery.

Laboratory Results

We specifically highlight lab results as a separate data type, because it creates a decision point in diagnostics and treatment. The test's description might include the following information:

Fluid or tissue	Characteristics
• Urine • Stool • Semen • Saliva • Sweat • Amniotic fluid • Pleural fluid • Exudate • Transudate and more • Blood	• Mass • Volume • Chemical components (blood glucose, electrolytes, enzymes, hormones, lipids, etc.) • Time stamp • Type of method (procedure used for the test) • Time aspect (interval of time for observation or measurement) and more

Medical Imaging (Fig. 8.15)

Another huge, complex and distinct data type is medical imaging, where visual information varies across modalities and can be presented in 2D or 3D formats:

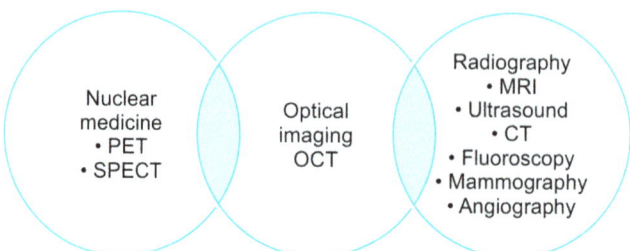

Fig. 8.15: Types of imaging.

Additionally, the majority of the aforementioned modalities can be used to extract quantitative imaging biomarkers, or QIBs. QIBs are able to help in the diagnosis, staging, treatment, and monitoring of a wide range of disorders since they reflect underlying physiological or biophysical processes on medical pictures. Numerous studies demonstrate the value of quantitative imaging biomarkers for non-invasive patient screening even though they have not yet been widely used in either research or clinical contexts.

Inpatient Health Monitoring

For care settings including anesthesia, the PACU, the NICU, critical care, and emergency care, inpatient health monitoring entails continuous data collection. A variety of vitals can be measured and tracked during the procedure thanks to specific monitoring technology, including:
- Pulse rate
- Pulse oximetry
- Metabolic and gas exchange
- Temperature
- Total hemoglobin
- Arrhythmia analysis
- Cardiac status
- Anesthesia parameters, such as entropy and NMT
- Data extraction

The two primary sources of data for the healthcare information system are managerial and clinical. They are conceptually kept in two different databases. However, data from both sources may be used by managers as well as clinician.

Purpose of Data Extraction

Certain specified data are collected from the database during the data extraction process and compiled for analysis. By using a data extraction tool, either a programmer or any user can complete this task as a database query (application). In order to choose certain data from any area of the database and organize or list them, a query is a programming script written in data query language (such as SQL).

Data that is being extracted could be:
- Confined to that of a single entity (a patient or any other entity)
- Belong to a group of entities

Data of a Single Entity

The patient is the entity in HIS that clinicians are most interested in. However, information on other entities like service units, employees, capital equipment, and consumables would also be of relevance to managers at all levels.

Data on a particular entity are taken out to demonstrate:
- The changes in qualities (properties, results, and so on) through time
- The measures performed (tasks, interventions, chronology of events)
- The things that occurred (incidents)

Data of a Group of Entities

Data from a group of entities is extracted and processed for managerial supervision, audit, and research purposes in order to provide an insight about the similarities or differences between group members. The group may consist of every entity, (i.e., population) present in the database. Frequently, only a portion of that population is being examined. Making registers, such as the hospital birth registry, from subsets of the complete population is one of the fundamental goals of data extraction. Clinicians frequently have an interest in researching a group of patients who have been chosen based on a variety of factors, including diagnosis, presentation, severity, or the kind of treatment received.

DATA ANALYSIS

Analysis refers to the act of **Figure 8.16**.
- Computation
- Categorization
- Comparison
- Manipulation

Using Information in Healthcare Management

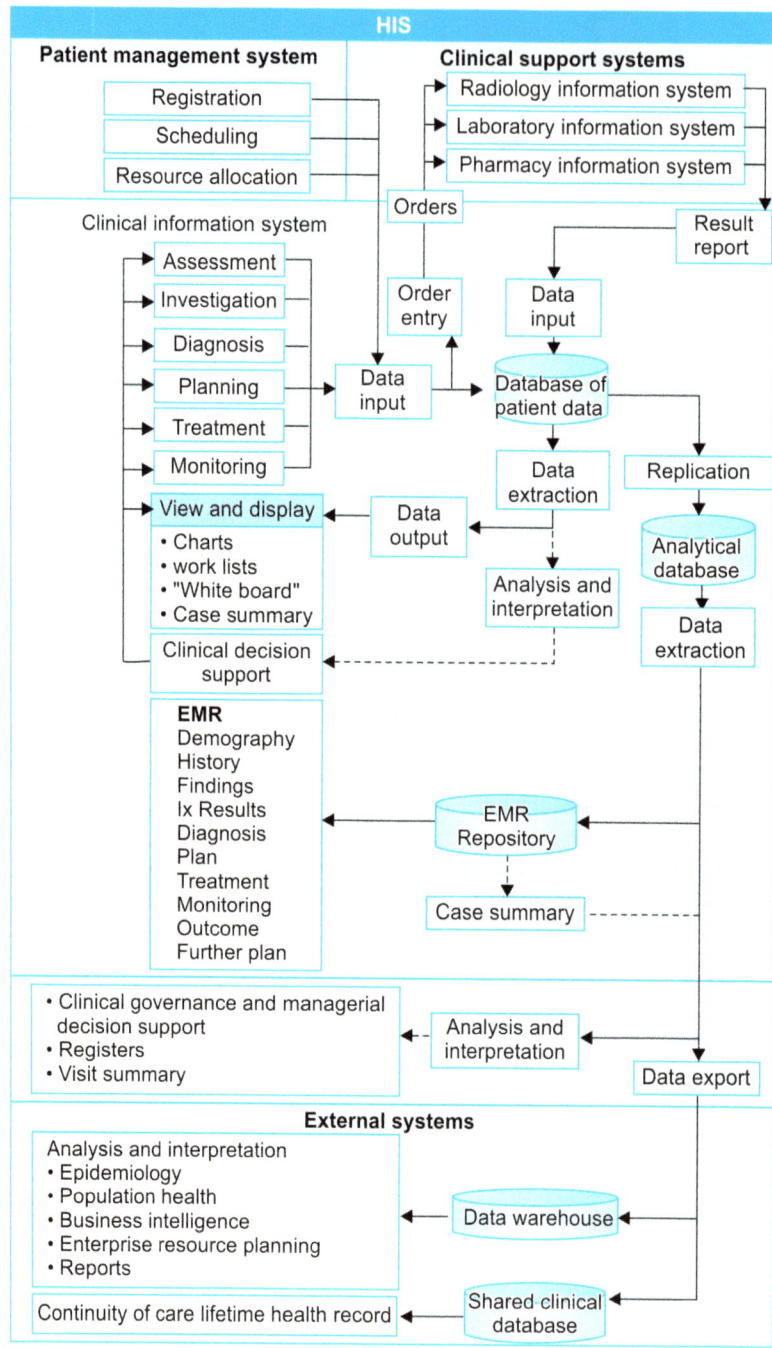

Fig. 8.16: System architecture of data analytics in hospital information system.

Using Information in Healthcare Management

DATA INTERPRETATION (FIG. 8.17)

Data that is analyzed is easier to interpret than raw data. Interpretation refers to the activity of using various means to reach a conclusion. These means include:
- Comparison
- Inference
- Projection

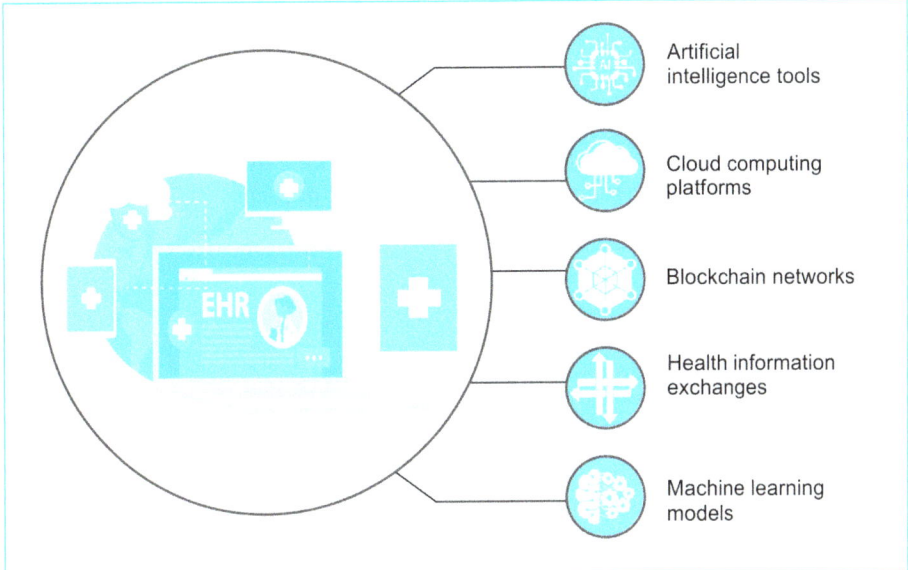

Fig. 8.17: Five types of healthcare data analytics technologies.

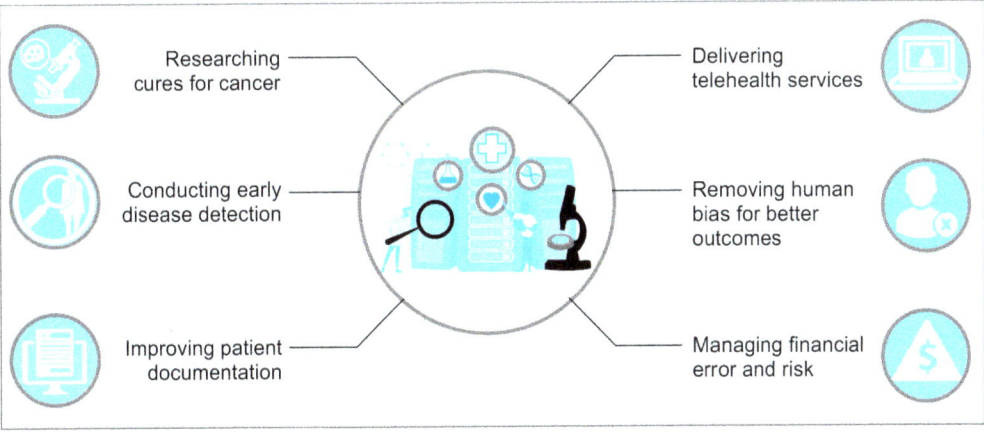

Fig. 8.18: Six real-world applications of healthcare data analytics.

Various Other Applications (Fig. 8.18)

- **Data mining:** It helps to discover patterns and trends in patient health data allowing to define underlying processes leading to diseases, such as recurrent episodes of skin rash, stomachache, hypertension, etc.
- **Text mining:** This technique allows finding patterns and trends indirectly, by extracting quantitative parameters from unstructured text data–such as EHR entries in free text.
- **Online analytical processing (OLAP):** OLAP is a set of tools allowing providers to analyze data in multiple dimensions simultaneously because it deals with preaggregated datasets. Online analytical processing uses three types of operations:

HEALTHCARE DATA IN DECISION MAKING

Data-based decision making (DBDM) is a method for making decisions based on verifiable facts and statistics at each stage of the problem-solving process (data). The effectiveness of the data's analysis and interpretation will determine whether the data-based approach is successful **(Fig. 8.19)**.

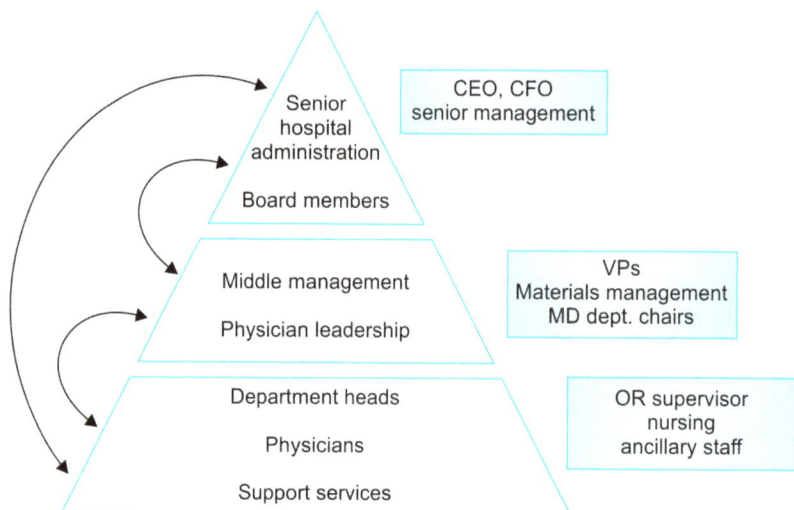

Fig. 8.19: Hospital decisions pathways.

VARIOUS APPROACHES TO DECISION MAKING

In general, by weighing several options and selecting the optimal course of action, the decision-making process aids hospital managers and administrators in resolving issues or challenges **(Fig. 8.20)**.

Making careful, well-informed judgments that will support the hospital's short- and long-term objectives is effective when done step-by-step.

Support for Clinical Judgment

Evidence-based medicine and diagnosis support are two approaches that are available to physicians in this situation and can be employed alone or jointly. Evidence-based medicine is used to determine the best course of treatment for each patient as well as to anticipate and minimize potential exacerbation, complication, and readmission risks. It is driven by insights gleaned from health data (mostly diagnosis, procedure, and treatment).

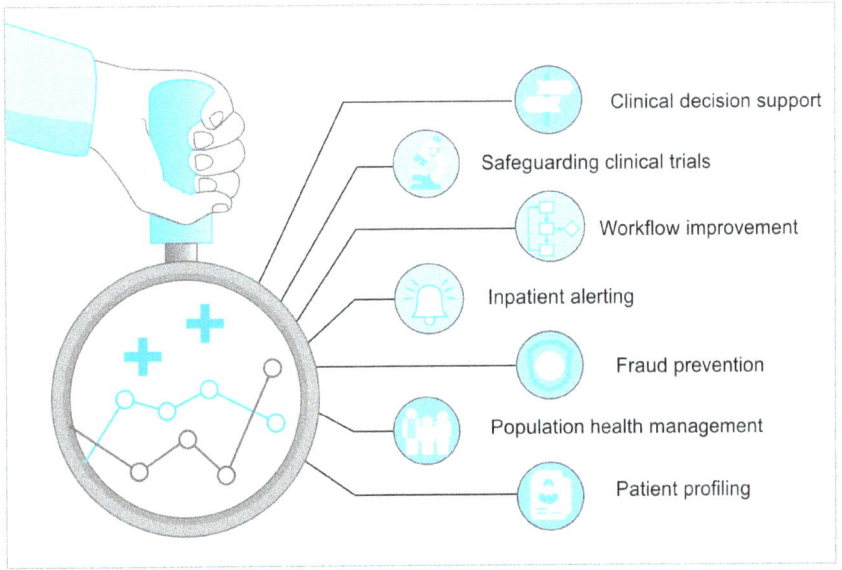

Fig. 8.20: Various measures to decision making in healthcare settings.

To suggest potential illnesses and perform procedures to confirm the disease, diagnosis support analyzes symptoms, test data, and patient history information. This helps to ensure prompt treatment, a reasonable length of stay, and favorable health outcomes.

Safeguarding Clinical Trials

Patient health data can be used to analyze existing clinical trials to improve trial design and eligible patient finding. Providers can match prospective treatment with fitting patients better, reducing trial failures and negative health outcomes.

Workflow Optimization

Health data analytics are used by quality insurance teams to assess performance, better understand clinical procedures, and locate care quality bottlenecks. They start process improvement activities by using information regarding procedures, primary and secondary diagnoses, and lab tests. They then keep an eye on current projects and their effectiveness to ensure lasting changes. For instance, an increase in C-sections may be entirely reasonable or needless and stem from a simple coincidence. In order to avoid unnecessary surgeries, healthcare professionals might examine data regarding each patient's justification for starting a C-section to see whether they need to intervene or revise the process.

Patient Notification

For inpatient settings and the care areas we established for the inpatient monitoring section, alerting caregivers to changes in patient health status is essential. Systems for collecting vital signs continuously analyze incoming data and alert medical professionals to good and negative trends, crucial dips, and peaks to ensure that surgery, post-surgical recovery, and other rehabilitation processes go without a hitch.

Fraud Mitigation

On a pre-adjudication basis, healthcare organizations can reduce inappropriate billing and avoid false or fraudulent claims without endangering their reputation or finances. To do this, trends indicating fraud or other abnormalities that lead to waste and abuse are found by analysing transaction data with claims and billing records. According to Mike Cottle, et al. (Transforming healthcare through big data), transaction data analytics with fraud detection capabilities helped CMS recover $3 billion.

Population Health Management

Although there are many ways to use data analytics to improve population health, researchers mostly focus on two areas: disease surveillance and chronic disease management.

As part of disease surveillance, healthcare professionals track diagnoses over time to identify disease outbreaks and ensure quick reaction to them.

One of the most crucial objectives in population health is the management of chronic diseases, particularly in terms of lowering hospital readmissions. In this situation, PGHD data analytics helps to follow patients' health state over time outside of a hospital or clinic so that doctors can start prompt interventions and prevent exacerbations, problems, and hospitalizations.

Patient Profiling

Health data analytics, according to McKinsey researchers, is useful for patient outreach. In order to identify patients with high health risks, identify those who require specific services or procedures, and identify those who do not, providers can apply advanced analysis (such as segmentation and predictive modeling) to patient profiles. With this useful information, providers can use proactive care options for individuals.

CHALLENGES IN HEALTHCARE DATA ANALYTICS (FIG. 8.21)

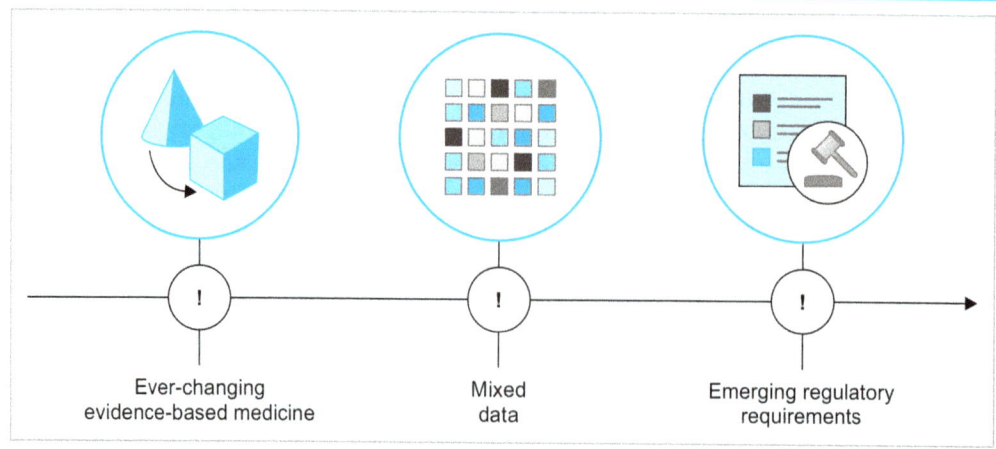

Fig. 8.21: Various challenges in healthcare data analytics.

Evidence-based Medicine

The accepted information about patient vitals and care delivery is continuously being updated by health professionals, therefore the understanding of targeting, measuring, and monitoring goals is evolving. For instance, the American diabetes association (ADA) regularly updates the standards of medical care in diabetes, adding new guidelines for prediabetes and hypoglycemia as well as modifying the nomenclature and care recommendations for diabetes to take into account the latest findings from clinical trials. Caretakers must therefore equip their data analytics programmes with the ability to process patient health data in accordance with industry-wide upgrades.

Mixed Data

All data are not created equal, and health data are anything but consistent. Information quality differs when it comes from various facilities, systems, devices, and sources. Furthermore, several methods might be used to capture the same piece of data in a single system, like an EHR. For instance, a diagnosis may be recorded in the clinical narrative, medical history, issue list for the patient, billing data, and other sources.

As a result, medical professionals occasionally enter data in free text, occasionally check boxes, and occasionally fill out drop-down lists in the fields, (e.g., in the clinical narrative). As a result, a mountain of structured and unstructured data is amassed, which should initially be handled differently but ultimately be standardized.

Emerging Regulatory Requirements

Regulatory requirements and reporting standards will also increase and evolve, especially since pay-for-performance approach gets broader adoption overtime and entails higher transparency in quality and pricing information. Accordingly, CMS will look into updating certain benchmarks and incentives, some of them will be reworked eventually. These changes are only adding to the reporting and analyzing burden for healthcare organizations from ACOs to private practices.

SUMMARY

A person who desires to play a significant role in healthcare without having direct patient contact may be interested in healthcare management. To be an integral member of the medical sector, one need not be in the operating room, dispense medicine, or provide direct care to patients. Without an efficient healthcare management system, a healthcare institution would be unable to provide effective patient care, retain qualified personnel, or generate a profit. Here is helpful information on healthcare administration. Prior to the introduction of fast improving medical technology, physicians had less need for healthcare administrators. However, the near-continuous development of medical technology (including changes in healthcare data systems) and regular changes in healthcare-related laws and regulations necessitate that hospitals and other medical centers employ specialists in these fields to ensure that everything operates as intended. Healthcare administration is just what its name says. It is the administration of a healthcare institution, such as a hospital or clinic. A healthcare manager is responsible for ensuring that a healthcare institution is operating properly in terms of budget, practitioners' objectives, and community requirements. A person in charge of healthcare management supervises the facility's day-to-day operations. This individual also serves as a spokesman when presenting journalists with information. The individual in charge of healthcare administration communicates with medical staff leaders on topics, such as medical equipment, department budgets, creating strategies to guarantee the institution fulfills its objectives, and maintaining a positive rapport with physicians, nurses, and other department heads. In addition to making choices about performance evaluations, staff expectations, budgeting, social media updates, and billing, the healthcare manager also takes decisions regarding performance evaluations, budgeting, social media updates, and billing.

REVIEW QUESTION

1. Define nursing information system.
2. Discuss briefly case management system.
3. What is patient classification system?
4. What nursing skills are needed for NIS?
5. Define data analytics.
6. What are the types of data analysis?
7. Enlist the steps of data management process.
8. What are the applications of data analytics?
9. Discuss about the components of nursing information system.
10. Enumerate the purposes of nursing information system.
11. Discuss about data management and data analytics.
12. Elaborate healthcare data usage in clinical decision making.

MULTIPLE CHOICE QUESTIONS

1. **The focus of data analysis is to:**
   a. Collect data from various sources
   b. Evaluate data for efficiency
   c. Identify data sources for later inclusion
   d. Transform data into a usable form.

2. **A downtime of the electronic health record (EHR) system is planned for three months from today. The informatics nurse is formulating a communication plan for the clinical staff about the downtime. The nurse plans to:**
   a. Announce the upcoming downtime at system-wide meetings, and at department meetings of specific system hospitals affected by the downtime
   b. Bring copies of the communication plan to IT meetings, and discuss it with the IT directors and managers
   c. Present the information at the super-user meetings, department and unit meetings, and at other specialty clinician meetings, in addition to having a message posted on the message-of-the-day screen in the EHR
   d. Print fliers with the downtime plan and post them in bathrooms and breakrooms, as well as on bulletin boards in various locations in the hospitals

3. **Integrating clinical practice guidelines with an electronic health record facilitates quality improvement measurement by:**
   a. Comparing guideline parameters to clinical outcomes
   b. Presenting results at the point of treatment decisions
   c. Providing reference information to measurement staff
   d. Representing patient acuity data.

Using Information in Healthcare Management

4. The combination of nursing, information and computer science to manage and process data into knowledge to use in nursing practice is called as:
   a. Hospital information system
   b. Management information system
   c. Nursing information system
   d. Patient in information system

5. Which component of nursing information system offers support for using pre-defined nursing terminologies and nursing classification such as NANDA, NIC and NOC?
   a. Case management system
   b. Nursing documentation system
   c. Clinical pathways
   d. Patient record system

6. Some of the following skills needed by nurse related to information system, *except*:
   a. Adapt the use of technologies to meet patient needs
   b. Teach patients about healthcare technologies
   c. Use information technologies to enhance one's own knowledge base.
   d. Controls the operating system with use of various operators

7. The science of analyzing raw data to make conclusions and interpretations about the information collected through various information systems is known as:
   a. Data integeration
   b. Data formation
   c. Data analytics
   d. Data management

8. Which analytics allows providers to focus on current clinical issues and look into the reasons of improved or decreased outcomes?
   a. Descriptive analysis
   b. Predictive analysis
   c. Ad hoc analysis
   d. Prescriptive analysis

9. Medical data can be classified as:
   a. Static, dynamic, occasional
   b. Static, dynamic, episodic
   c. Dynamic, static, logical
   d. Logical, descriptive, static

10. Which of the following is not application of data analytics?
    a. Data mining
    b. Text mining
    c. Decision support
    d. Support services

Answer Key

1. d	2. c	3. a	4. c	5. b
6. d	7. c	8. a	9. b	10. d

CHAPTER 9

Information Law and Governance in Clinical Practice

> **At the end of this chapter, student will able to learn about:**
> ❖ Ethical legal issues in healthcare informatics
> ❖ Purposes for the code of ethics
> ❖ Ethics resources used in health informatics
> ❖ Ethical legal issues related to digital health applied to nursing

TERMINOLOGIES

- **Confidentiality:** This relates to the capability of protecting data in the EHR system so that only authorized individuals can access it.
- **Integrity:** Integrity is the ability to maintain the original representation of data despite any modifications.
- **Malpractice:** The failure of a nurse to perform in accordance with the expected standard of practice is known as nursing malpractice.
- **Negligence:** A healthcare provider's conduct or omission that differs from the accepted standards of care and causes harm to the patient is referred to as nursing negligence.
- **Autonomy:** The right to self-determination is a fundamental human right that all people possess.
- **Justice and equality:** Everyone has the right to be treated fairly because they are all created equal.
- **Beneficence:** It states that everyone has a responsibility to further the interests of others when doing so is consistent with the affected party's core moral principles.
- **Non-malfeasance:** It states that everyone has a responsibility to stop people from hurting one other when they are able to do so without causing themselves undue harm.
- **Impossibility:** All rights and obligations are subject to the requirement that they can be fulfilled in light of the current situation.

INTRODUCTION

Research and practice in the health professions should be guided by human values. Like other health professions, healthcare informatics addresses questions of proper and improper conduct, honorable and dishonorable deeds, and right and wrong.

Examining the moral foundations and ethical issues surrounding their study and practice is a responsibility shared by students and practitioners of the health sciences, including informatics. The main difficulties are generally well understood, despite the fact that ethical questions in medical, nursing, human subjects research, psychology, social work, and related professions continue to change. Major bioethical issues have been discussed in a variety of academic, professional, and pedagogical settings. Despite some of them receiving attention for decades, ethical issues in health informatics are generally less well-known.

People frequently believe that the privacy of patient data kept electronically is the main area of informatics ethics concern. The use of informatics tools in clinical settings, the choice of who should use them, the function of system evaluation, the duties of system developers, maintainers, and vendors, and the use of computers to track clinical outcomes in order to guide future practice are just a few of the other ethical issues that the field faces, despite the importance and significance of confidentiality and privacy. Additionally, informatics raises numerous crucial legal and regulatory issues.

ETHICAL LEGAL ISSUES IN HEALTHCARE INFORMATICS

According to the Code of Ethics, "the ethical responsibilities of the health information management (HIM) professional include safeguarding the privacy and security of health information; disclosing health information; developing, using, and maintaining health information systems; and ensuring the accessibility and integrity of health information."

It also gives seven purposes for the code of ethics:
1. The support of best practices in health information management.
2. The mission of health information management's fundamental values being identified.
3. A list of the major moral tenets that represent the fundamental virtues.
4. Establishing moral standards that serve as a guide for decisions and behaviors.
5. Creation of a framework for professional conflict resolution and ethical uncertainty clarification.
6. Establishing moral guidelines that enable the general public to hold health information management experts responsible.
7. Presenting chances for mentors to lead novice practitioners in ethical instruction.

The application of ethical principles to the field of health informatics is known as ethics in health informatics or health informatics ethics. Health informatics essentially consists of three components: software, information, and healthcare. Systems of information are created to make it easier to provide healthcare or carry out related tasks. Processing information effectively is another topic covered in health informatics. A significant amount of patient data must be archived and available for retrieval at any time. Information transfer between healthcare organizations must be managed securely. Software is ultimately responsible for processing, storing, and retrieving information. In fact, software solutions are required to handle clinics, hospitals, and the data that larger healthcare providers require.

Information Law and Governance in Clinical Practice

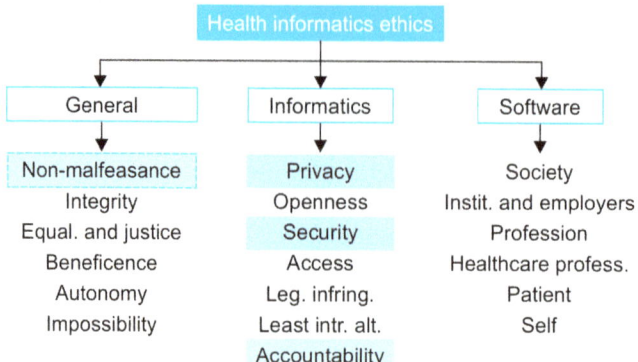

Fig. 9.1: Aspects of health informatics ethics.

Informatics Ethics Covers Seven Principles

- **Privacy:** Every person has a fundamental right to privacy, which includes control over how their personal data is collected, stored, accessed, used, communicated, manipulated, and disposed of.
- **Principle of transparency:** Personal data subjects must be informed appropriately and promptly about the collection, storage, access, use, transmission, manipulation, and disposal of their data.
- **Principle of access:** The owner of a health record has the right to access it and the right to have it updated with regard to accuracy, completeness, and applicability.
- **Legitimate infringement principle:** The only limitations on the fundamental right to control the collection, storage, access, use, manipulation, communication, and disposition of personal data are the legitimate, appropriate, and relevant data needs of a free, responsible, and democratic society, as well as the equal and competing rights of other people.
- **Least intrusive alternative principle:** Any violation of an individual's privacy rights, as well as that person's right to control over person-related data, may only take place in a way that is least intrusive and interferes the least with that individual's rights.
- **Principle of accountability:** Any violation of a person's right to privacy and their ability to control their personal information must be properly disclosed to the affected party in a timely manner.
- **Principle of security:** Data that has been legitimately obtained about a person must be protected from loss, degradation, illegal destruction, access, use, manipulation, alteration, and communication by taking all reasonable and necessary safeguards.

ETHICS RESOURCES USED IN HEALTH INFORMATICS

There are many ethical resources available, including codes of ethics, case studies, ethics committees and personnel, as well as informal dialogues, to assist in resolving such dilemmas and providing answers to the difficult topics. These tools aid in choosing the best course of action.

- **Codes of conduct:** Ethics codes are official texts that outline ethical obligations. Members of the profession or organization are expected to uphold the ethical standards set forth in these codes. These regulations also correct any erroneous assumptions regarding ethical standards

- **A case study:** There are frequently references to earlier ethical disputes and circumstances that may have been addressed in a particular way. These decisions can be used as precedent.
- **Assistants and ethics committees:** Committees and trained personnel can be used by organizations to explore and resolve ethical problems. These might include ethics committees or experts in ethics who are consulted when ethical dilemmas arise.
- **Informal conversations:** Conversations with friends or coworkers can result in informal advice about how to settle an ethical conflict. We focus on the application of codes of ethics in the setting of this study. We take this action since ethics codes offer a more official structure.

ETHICAL LEGAL ISSUES RELATED TO DIGITAL HEALTH APPLIED TO NURSING

Digital health technologies have permeated every part of our life thanks to technological advancements and breakthroughs in Internet connectivity. A growing number of digital health technologies, such as hospital information systems, electronic health records, e-Prescriptions, e-Referrals, personal digital assistants, wearable, telemedicine, and tele-monitoring, make it easier to store, transmit, and retrieve medical data, enhance patient-provider communication, track biological and physiological parameters, and provide remote health and social services. However, the use of technology in health and social care services also raises certain concerns about the level of ethical behavior that should be expected from those who create digital health technologies. New technologies in the health and social care sectors raise ethical concerns about things like privacy, security, equity, accessibility, and data protection. Determining what defines ethics and which codes of ethics to follow will be a challenge for anyone involved in the design, development, and deployment of digital health technology and apps. To deal with the effects of digital technologies on our societies, numerous frameworks and rules have been formed. To handle significant engineering ethics-related software needs, requirement engineers must follow the relevant codes of ethics.

For electronic health records, privacy and confidentiality, security, and data integrity and availability are the top three ethical considerations.

- **Privacy and confidentiality:** "The right to privacy" refers to "the demand of individuals to be left alone, from surveillance or intervention from other persons, organizations, or the government. As a result of a clinical engagement, information is disclosed that is deemed confidential and needs to be kept secure. The data may include identity information, diagnoses, treatment and progress notes, and laboratory findings. It may also be kept in a variety of formats, (e.g., paper, video, electronic files). This category does not include data that cannot be used to determine the patient's name, such as the quantity of men with prostate cancer treated at a particular facility. Only with the patient's consent or as permitted by law may patient information be disclosed to third parties. This does not imply, however, that doctors cannot access patient data. Without the patient's consent, information may be disclosed for administrative, financial, or therapeutic objectives. The patient also has legal, federal, and state-granted rights to see his or her health record, get a copy of it, and make changes to it. Making sure that information is only accessible to those who are authorized is essential to maintaining confidentiality. Authorizing users is the first step in the process of restricting access—limiting who can see what. The practice administrator, for instance, identifies the users, decides what degree of information is required, and gives usernames and passwords in a medical practice. Basic requirements for passwords include mandating them to be changed at predetermined intervals, establishing a minimum character count, and outlawing password reuse. Many businesses and medical practices use a two-tier authentication system that includes a biometric identifier scan, such as a face, palm, finger, or retinal scan.

- **Security:** The rise of EHRs, increased use of mobile devices like smartphones, medical identity theft, and the eagerly anticipated data exchange between and among organizations, clinicians, federal agencies, and patients are all contributing factors to the growing concern over the security of health information. Patients might not be honest with the doctor if their trust has been damaged. Records in the office must be safeguarded if the patient is to trust the clinician. The security procedures required to safeguard patient information and practice data must be known to medical staff. Data manipulation, destruction, and hacking are additional potential threats, so all users must be included in security measures and ongoing training programmes. Firewalls, antivirus software, and intrusion detection software are a few security techniques that safeguard data integrity. No matter the method employed, a complete security programme and an audit trail system must be in effect to ensure the integrity of the data. Providers and organizations are required to formally name a security officer to work with a group of health IT specialists who can inventory the system's users and technologies, identify security flaws and threats, assign a risk or likelihood of security concerns in the organization, and address those concerns. One of the staff members working in the doctor's office can be given the duties related to privacy and security, or they can be outsourced.

- **Integrity and availability:** Integrity guarantees that the data is true and unaltered. Given that data transmission across systems is increasingly widespread in the healthcare sector; this is a general word for a crucial notion in the electronic environment. In ambulatory offices, hospitals, rehabilitation facilities, and other settings across the continuum of care, data may be gathered and used in a variety of systems. As it flows between and among systems, this data may be mistakenly or purposely altered. Documentation flaws or a lack of proper documentation integrity can also lead to poor data integrity. The data can become useless if the system is breached or inundated with requests. Electronic health record systems frequently feature redundant components, also known as fault-tolerance systems, to ensure availability, so if one component fails or encounters issues, the system will move to a backup component.

SUMMARY

The more significant specific ethical obligations and rights that result from these Principles of Informatics Ethics are described in the Code of Ethics for Health Informatics Professionals. It should be highlighted that the Code, like any code of ethical behavior, can only serve as a guide. The specifics of the relevant circumstance will determine how each provision of the Code will apply in a given case and the nature of any specific ethical rights or obligations that are involved. The most difficult challenges in our increasingly data-driven culture are privacy and security. EHRs are utilized by patients, doctors, and other healthcare workers more frequently due to a number of benefits, but they also present a number of privacy, security, and integrity issues. By taking into account the elements and difficulties of e-health services, our main contribution to this paper is to present state-of-the-art approaches for security, privacy, and integrity aspects of EHS. The assessment identifies numerous potential and difficulties for enhancing privacy and security safeguards in the future and finds that the effectiveness of electronic health records is significantly impacted by getting privacy and security correctly.

REVIEW QUESTION

1. Explain the ethical legal issues in healthcare informatics.
2. Explain the purposes for the code of ethics in healthcare information.
3. Explain the ethical legal issues related to digital health applied to nursing.

MULTIPLE CHOICE QUESTIONS

1. The nurse's involvement in an ethical scenario is taken into consideration is called_____.
   a. Agitator
   b. Moral
   c. Dignity
   d. Humor

2. _____ is a legal instrument that enables a person to provide the public with specific skills and expertise.
   a. Law
   b. Error
   c. License
   d. Scope of practice

3. Professional nurse accountable to the following, *except*:
   a. To clients
   b. To code of ethics
   c. To self
   d. To the profession

Answer Key
1. b   2. d   3. c

CHAPTER 10

Healthcare Quality and Evidence-based Practice

> **At the end of this chapter, student will able to learn about:**
> ❖ Evidence-based practice
> ❖ Differences between evidence-based practice and quality improvement
> ❖ Role of nurse in quality improvement through EBP
> ❖ Purposes of health informatics standards
> ❖ Healthcare data standards
> ❖ Development of healthcare standards

TERMINOLOGIES

- **Quality healthcare:** Providing high-quality healthcare increases the likelihood of achieving targeted health outcomes and is in line with professional consensus.
- **Evidence-based practice:** The definition of evidence-based practise is the integration of the most recent research findings with clinical knowledge and patient values to improve healthcare outcomes.
- **Evidence-based medicine:** It is "the conscious, explicit, and prudent use of current best evidence in choices concerning the care of individual patients."
- **Evidence-based quality improvement:** It is when evidence-based procedures are modified to better suit local needs and increase the acceptance and efficacy of various healthcare innovations.
- **Quality improvement:** In order to achieve the adjustments that will improve patient outcomes (health), system performance (care), and professional growth, everyone — including healthcare professionals, patients, and their families—must work together and continuously to improve quality.
- **Standards:** Through a collaborative process involving the audience that will be using the standards, standards development organizations (SDOs) establish, revise, and maintain standards.
- **Healthcare standards:** A document that outlines rules, guidelines, or characteristics for actions or their outcomes in the fields of information for health and health information and communications technology. It is established based on evidence, by consensus, and is approved by an established body.

EVIDENCE-BASED QUALITY IMPROVEMENT

Introduction

Evidence bases must be established for the actual implementation plans for evidence-based medicine. Evidence-based quality improvement refers to the use of implementation techniques that are supported by research (EBQI). Evidence-based implementation strategies include tailoring to the local context, using a quality manager, regular data collection to drive and evaluate change, and performance feedback, leadership support, external and internal facilitation (also known as a clinical champion), provider and patient education. The most effective EBQI occurs when researchers, clinicians, and clinic leadership work together as true partners. Clinicians and administrators give the specialized expertize required to adapt evidence-based practise to their unique organizational demands.

One of the most frequently used concepts in healthcare and health systems is evidence-based medicine. Another is quality improvement. One of the biggest medical breakthroughs of the 20th century is evidence-based medicine, which has influenced fields far outside medicine, such as "evidence-based policy" and "evidence-based conservation."

Comparing quality improvement with evidence-based medicine may offer insights to guide the future development of the quality improvement movement, as there is growing interest in integrating quality improvement into routine clinical practise.

Definition

It is a "multilevel, stakeholder-driven approach to continuous quality improvement, evidence-based quality improvement (EBQI) makes use of leadership involvement, formative data feedback, quality improvement training, measurement-based improvement, and external facilitation to promote implementation".

"EBP mandates that decisions regarding medical treatment be supported by the best accessible, current, valid, and pertinent evidence. These choices should be made by persons who are receiving care, guided by the implicit and explicit knowledge of those who are giving care, and taking into account the resources that are available".

Information from electronic health records, hospital databases, and other datasets is used for rigorous research and quality assessment exercises that contribute to improvements in patient care. This process is aided by the dissemination of information to clinicians, researchers, and quality leaders as well as by the execution of quality improvement initiatives.

Competencies of Healthcare Professionals for EBQI

- **Provide patient-centered care:** Which entails recognizing, respecting, and caring for patients' differences, values, preferences, and expressed needs; easing pain and suffering; coordinating ongoing care; listening to, clearly informing, communicating with, and educating patients; sharing decision-making and management; and persistently advocating disease prevention, wellness, and the promotion of healthy lifestyles, with an emphasis on population health.
- **Work in interdisciplinary teams:** Assemble interdisciplinary teams and interact, communicate, and integrate care to guarantee consistent and dependable care.
- **Employ evidence-based practice:** Use evidence-based practise; for the best care, combine the best research with clinical knowledge and patient values; and, to the extent practical, take part in learning and research activities.

- **Use quality improvement techniques:** Recognize errors and hazards in care; comprehend and put into practise fundamental safety design principles, such as standardization and simplification; continuously understand and measure the quality of care in terms of structure, process, and outcomes in relation to patient and community needs; and design and test interventions to alter processes and systems of care with the aim of improving quality.
- **Utilize informatics:** Communicate, manage knowledge, mitigate error, and support decision making using information technology.

Differences between Evidence-based practice and Quality Improvement

Evidence-based practice	Quality improvement
A continuous method of clinical practise that incorporates a thorough review, evaluation, and synthesis of pertinent literature, clinical knowledge, and patient preferences and values	The constant and collaborative efforts of everyone—healthcare professionals, patients, payers, planners, educators—to bring forth improvements that will improve patient outcomes, system performance, and professional growth
To converting information with the intention of improving practise	Transferring knowledge with the intention of enhancing application
Transforming the data into phrases for use in clinical decision-making	In most cases, comprehensive critical analysis and in-depth literature studies are not necessary for QI
Finding and incorporating the best available evidence into clinical practise requires innovation in EBP	Based on site-specific and results aren't meant to provide knowledge that can be applied generally or the strongest proof

Quality of Care

The possibility that intended health outcomes will occur as a result of individual and population health interventions is referred to as quality of care. It is crucial for establishing universal health coverage and is based on professional knowledge supported by evidence. It is crucial to carefully assess the quality of care and health services as nations make commitments to achieving Health for All. Although there are various ways to describe great health care, it is becoming increasingly recognized that quality services should include the following:

- **Effective:** Offering people who require it evidence-based healthcare services.
- **Safe:** It means keeping the individuals for whom the care is designed safe.
- **People-centered:** Care that is focused on the needs, values, and preferences of the individual.
- **Timely:** Reducing wait times and occasionally damaging delays.
- **Equitable:** Care that is provided in an equitable manner does not differ in quality based on a patient's gender, ethnicity, region, or socioeconomic situation.
- **Integrated:** Providing care that makes the complete spectrum of health services available throughout the life course is known as integrated care.
- **Efficiency:** It means making the most of the resources at hand and minimizing waste.

ROLE OF NURSE IN QUALITY IMPROVEMENT THROUGH EBP

❑ Healthcare providers may harness the power of data. The usefulness of data for decision-making and giving the correct information to the right person at the right time is something that nurses and other healthcare professionals are discovering today.
❑ Technology and informatics continue to expand the toolkit for patient care, but there are still obstacles to overcome, such as creating and using efficient risk assessment models, standardizing user interfaces and functionality, creating and implementing safety-related decision support, and establishing social norms and legal frameworks for sharing patient data.
❑ Health information technology (HIT) is a tool used by clinicians in evidence-based practise (EBP) that promotes patient-centered decision-making, improves patient quality and safety, and links patients to community-based and other educational initiatives to improve health literacy. Health information from both patients and providers is combined and kept, shared, and evaluated.
❑ The electronic health record (EHR), patient portals, or personal health records are all examples of health information technology (HIT) (E-prescribing). To make health-related decision-making easier, the digital gap between patients and providers has been reduced.
❑ When patient-related data are combined, rich information is produced, which ultimately leads to more knowledge and understanding about patient care.
❑ The coupling of nursing informatics and EBP suggests the integration of an empathic, informed, and patient-centered method of practice.
❑ Nurses must be competent enough to use information technology and must have information literacy.

Therefore to utilize EBP through nursing information technology there should be separate nurse informatics innovator which should have the following roles **(Fig. 10.1)**:

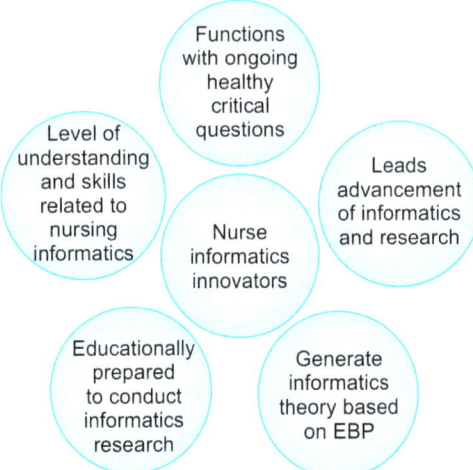

Fig. 10.1: Role of nurse informatics innovators.

HEALTHCARE DATA STANDARDS

Healthcare organizations communicate information in accordance with a set of standards, just like other sectors of the economy. Standards are accepted techniques for linking systems. Standards may be related to safety, data transmission, data structure or format, or the definitions of terms or codes.

By attempting to adopt standards whenever possible, healthcare businesses can lower implementation costs, quicken integration projects, and benefit from shared tooling. Data standards are created to ensure that all parties use the same language and the same approach to sharing, storing, and interpreting information. In healthcare, standards make up the backbone of interoperability—or the ability of health systems to exchange medical data regardless of domain or software provider.

The key to facilitating information sharing and communication between departments, health agencies, and health workers is standards. They are required for linking between systems through an apparent seamless integration of highly distributed systems, as well as for the information content, language, database, and system architectures. This is frequently described as "interoperability." To index and organize health-related information for quick retrieval and to gather uniform clinical data for research purposes, electronic medical or health records need standards. Without standards, classification, and coding systems, it is impossible to meaningfully compare the health status, healthcare procedures, expenditures, and results across different treatment modalities, health organizations, regions, or nations.

Definition

Standards: A standard is a set of rules, conditions, or specifications that govern how terms are defined, components are categorized, materials are specified, operations are carried out, procedures are defined, and quantity and quality are measured when describing materials, products, systems, services, or practises.

Healthcare standards: A document that establishes standards, guidelines, or characteristics for actions or their outcomes in the fields of health information and communications technology based on evidence, consensus, and approval by an established organization.

PURPOSES OF HEALTH INFORMATICS STANDARDS (FIG. 10.2)

In general, HI standards support clinical practise as well as the administration, provision, and assessment of healthcare services.
- To "promote interoperability between independent systems, to enable compatibility and uniformity for health information and data, as well as to avoid duplication of effort and redundancies.
- Semantic interoperability is the ability to interpret, and, therefore, to make effective use of the information so exchanged.
- In order to successfully transmit information and analyze and apply it, interoperability is required in all healthcare settings around the world.
- Easier manufacturing, supply, and trade are other significant objectives, as are reducing duplication of effort and redundancy.

Healthcare Quality and Evidence-based Practice

- The secure, efficient incorporation of ICT and information management into clinical practise.
- The fundamental goals of HI standards are to facilitate interoperability and to direct safe, efficient HI activity.

DEVELOPMENT OF HEALTHCARE STANDARDS

Step 1—Determine the needs of the firm: Stakeholders identify business needs and submit specifications for a standard to a standard development organization, or SDO, such as healthcare providers, hospitals, health insurance, or software suppliers.

Step 2—Workgroup collaboration: A team with clinicians, healthcare administrators, health information professionals, software developers, and specialists in regulatory requirements is tasked with creating a standard. The standard draught and the implementation plan are both created by the workgroup.

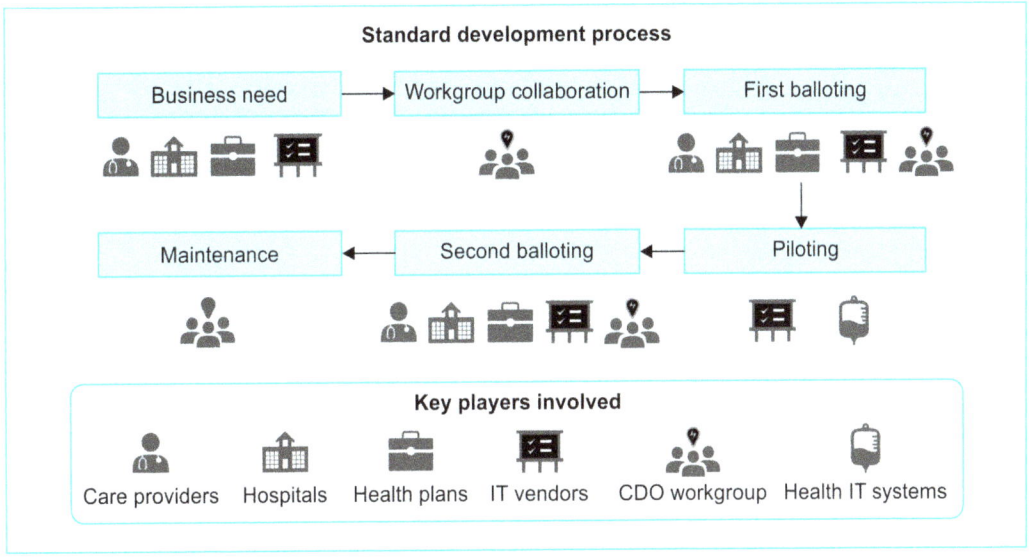

Fig. 10.2: Procedure of healthcare standard development.

Step 3—First balloting: Stakeholder comments on the draught are taken into consideration by the workgroup while creating the standards. All participants then cast their votes for the pilot-ready draught criteria.

Step 4—Piloting: Vendors of software and/or healthcare systems test the standards' draught version and offer input.

Step 5—Second balloting: The workgroup incorporates feedback from piloting and sends the draft for the second balloting. Upon receiving comments, the workgroup makes all necessary improvements. Finally, workgroup members and stakeholders vote to approve the draft as a normative standard for use.

Step 6—Implementation and maintenance: The SDO implements standards, fixes issues, and collects feedback to make improvements.

Key healthcare coding systems			
	Developer	Area of use	Key applications
ICD-10-CM	WHO	Diseases and diagnoses	Statistics billing
CPT	AMA	Medical procedures and services	Treatment tracking billing
HCPCS	CMS	Products, supplies, devices, and services not covered by CPT	Billing medicare and medicaid
CDT	ADA	Oral health and dental services	Documenting dental treatment
SNOMED CT	SNOMED international	Clinical terminology	Recording, aggregation, and sharing clinical data
LOINC	Regenstrief institute	Laboratory orders and results	Transmitting laboratory and test observations
NDC	FDA	Pharmacy products	Drug reimbursement reporting drugs and biological products
RxNorm	NLM	Clinical drugs and drug delivery devices	Recording and processing drug information

Fig. 10.3: Terminology standards used in healthcare.

SUMMARY

Evidence-based practice (EBP) has gained appeal as a transformational approach to healthcare during the last couple decades. Doctor of Nursing Practice (DNP)-educated nurses who apply EBP will examine the finest research data, link it to the patient's history, and then incorporate the patient's values into treatment. Implementing EBP has been shown to improve patient outcomes and save costs regardless of the institution or environment. In nursing, evidence-informed practice is a method that integrates the finest research, clinical experience, and patient feedback. The basis of this problem-solving strategy is straightforward: to deliver superior patient care. When improved patient outcomes are achieved, the advantages do not end there. As a result of including the patient in the dialogue and decision-making process, evidence-based practice increases openness and accountability. The method reduces the demand for healthcare resources and practitioners, resulting in cost savings.

REVIEW QUESTION

1. Define EBQI.
2. What is the difference between evidence-based practice and quality improvement?
3. Who is nurse informative innovator?

4. Define healthcare standards.
5. Define briefly ISO.
6. Elaborate the role of nurse in evidence-based quality improvement.
7. Discuss the process of healthcare standard.

MULTIPLE CHOICE QUESTIONS

1. What are the components of evidence-based practice?
    a. Expert opinion, research evidence, quantitative research and clinical trials
    b. Clinical expertise, research evidence, practice contexts and funders perspectives
    c. Research evidence, clinical expertise, patient values and information from practice contexts
    d. Patients perspective, expert opinion, research evidence and clinical expertise

2. Elements of quality management system are _____.
    a. Organizational structure   b. Responsibilities
    c. Procedures   d. All the three

3. What is the world body for standards formulation?
    a. WHO   b. ILO
    c. ISO   d. QC

4. The quality management strategy that expands on conventional quality assurance methods by placing an emphasis on the organization and systems
    a. Quality control   b. Quality design
    c. Continuous quality improvement d. Quality assurance

5. What is the role of the American Health Information Management Association?
    a. Serving as a clearinghouse for data collection and analysis in healthcare.
    b. Networking all IT staff for support of future trends.
    c. Providing education, certification, and support to HIM professionals.
    d. Founding scholarships for healthcare professionals working overseas.

6. Health information management is the department assigned to do which of the following?
    a. HIM creates and enforces budgets.
    b. HIM oversees the patients plan of care for the staff.
    c. HIM maintains the safe, secure, and confidential health record.
    d. HIM develops the processes for facility engineering safety.

7. There is no logical basis of making decision or taking action without the following:
    a. Knowledge   b. Quality
    c. Standard   d. Condition

8. Healthcare quality improvement defines when the attributes based on individual needs are one of the following:
    a. Advanced care   b. Patient centered care
    c. Evidence-based care   d. Modern healthcare

Answer Key
1. c   2. d   3. c   4. c   5. c
6. c   7. c   8. b

Index

Page numbers followed by *f* refer to figure.

A

Accelerate decision-making 10
Access support 10
Access tool 2
Accessibility toolbar 15
Accountability, principle of 130
Accuracy 2, 69
Administrative benefits 47
Administrative transactions 98
Admissions information 4
Adopting e-health, challenges in 99
Allied health professionals 47
Analytical domain 36, 41*f*
Application 100
    knowledge of 88
    server 36
    software 3
Artificial intelligence 29
    to data processing 68
Autofill 22
Automated chatbots and voice messages 67
Automation 2
Autonomy 128
Autosum 22

B

Beneficence 128
Better care planning 111
Better communication 69
Better governance 69
Better opportunities 4
Better workload functionality 111
Blockchain and future healthcare technology 68
Business operations 54

C

Capture, knowledge of 87
Care, quality of 136
Case management
    model 109*f*
    system for 109
Case studies 91, 131
Catastrophes, plan for 78
Cerner 32
Change theory 29
Charts 22
Clinical care 97
Clinical data integration 108, 108*f*
Clinical decision 103
    support, tools for 43
Clinical informatics 33
Clinical information system 42, 48-51
    benefits of 49
    components of 52*f*
Clinical judgment, support for 122
Clinical knowledge 85
Clinical pathway model 106*f*
Clinical practice, information law and
    governance in 128
Clinical procedure, transformation in 34
Clinical research 98
Clinical support services, system for 52, 52*f*
Cognitive theory 29
Collaboration 11
Common user-system interface 53
Communication 5
Comparing groups 9
Computer 1, 2
    application 1
    characteristics of 2
    components of 2
    databases 7
    in literature search and database,
        use of 6
    in nursing practice, use of 5
    in research, use of 5
    in teaching and learning, use of 3
Computerized generated data 115
Computerized physician order entry 115
Conduct, codes of 130
Confidentiality 128, 131
Consumer
    health 97
    inclinations 96
Convenient view 69
Cost effective 34
Customer relationship management 85

Index

D

Data 1
  analytics 103, 113
    system architecture of 120*f*
    types of 114
  classification of 115
  collection 9, 101
  export 11
  extraction 32
    purpose of 119
  import 11
  interpretation 121
  management 115, 116
  migration 65
  mining 122
  preparation 10
  privacy 65
  security 78
  source 115
  storage hardware 37
Database 37
  content and organizational structure 37
  creation 115
  domain 37*f*
  management system 38*f*, 53
  server 37
Decision making 85, 122
Decision support system 108*f*, 109
Digital health 95
Discovery
  analytics 114
  knowledge of 87
Dissemination 101
Document management system 32
Documenting nursing care 105*f*
Drug-related errors, reduction of 76

E

Easy communication 4
Easy information access 76
Education 28, 29
Effective patient care practices 78
E-health 95
  applications 97
  drivers of 96
  system 96
Electronic health record 42, 49, 62, 63, 66*f*, 71, 137
  adoption of 76
  features of 63*f*
  implementation 65
  standard 69
    goals of 67
  system 66
Electronic medical record 24, 32, 42, 49, 56, 60, 62
  benefits of 69
  software 32
Electronic record technology 67
Employ evidence-based practice 135
Encoding 85
Ensure adequate training 67
Ensure strong leadership 67
Enterprise risk management 73
E-prescription process 64*f*
E-records, patient information system on 63*f*
Ethical legal issues 129, 131
Ethics committees 131
Evidence-based medicine 125, 134
Evidence-based practice 134, 136, 140
Evidence-based quality improvement 134, 135
Excel
  features 22
  worksheet 20

F

Financial information system 50
Financial transactions 98
Fluid 117
Fraud mitigation 124
Future preparation 10

G

Gradual implementation 75
GraphPad prism 11

H

Hardware 2
Health 29
Health data 117
  management 29
Health informatics 26, 130
  ethics, aspects of 130*f*
  principle of 26
  standards 91
    purposes of 138
Health information
  governance 75
  management 32
  system 33, 60
  technology 26, 137
Health system policy 97

Index

Healthcare 32, 140*f*
   data 103, 122
      analysis of 113
      evaluation of 113
      generating sources in 116*f*
      presentation of 113
      standards 138
   data analytics 124*f*
      challenges in 124
      four types of 114*f*
      six real-world applications of 121*f*
      technologies, five types of 121*f*
   informatics 129
      systems 35, 42
   management 103
   professionals, competencies of 135
   quality 134
   research 29
   standards 134, 138
      development of 139, 139*f*
Hospital information system 43, 46, 74, 120*f*
   aims of 45
   benefits of 46
   classification of 51*f*
   communication flow 44*f*
   components 48*f*
   history of 46
   hybrid 35
   portal 55
   role of 54*f*
   subsystems of 47
Hospital management system 29, 45

I

Imaging, types of 118*f*
Implementation cost 65
Inadequate planning 66
Ineffective interoperability 66
Informal conversations 131
Informatics 33
Information 1
   storage 5
   system 32, 50, 53, 103
      architecture of 33
      role of 33
   technology 75, 112
      future of 76
   use of 97
Inpatient health monitoring 118
Integration 53, 69
Integrity 128, 132

Intensive care
   clinical information systems in 49
   units 48
Interdisciplinary team 66
Internet 5

J

Justice 128

K

Keypad 3
Knowledge 1
   and information in healthcare, applied
      examples of 29
   management system 86
      advantages of 88
      challenges of 88
      components of 87
      dimensions of 86

L

Laboratory information system 50
Learning, better rate of 4
Least intrusive alternative principle 130
Legitimate infringement principle 130
Literature search 6
Login and searching in system 56
Losing data, chances of 28

M

Malpractice 128
Management system 53
Managerial decision support systems 54
Managerial information system 55*f*
   components of 54
Master patient index 43
Medical errors, avoiding of 34
Medical history 65
Medical imaging 118
Medication administration 111
Medicine
   digital imaging and communications in 47
   systematized nomenclature of 92
M-health 95
Microsoft
   excel 12, 20
   office 2010 12, 13
   PowerPoint 22
   word 2010 12, 14, 16

Index

Minitab 11
Mobility 5
Mouse 3, 17

N

Nanotechnology 29
Negligence 128
Network architecture 39
New systems 74
North American Nursing Diagnosis Association 104
Nurse informatics innovators, role of 137f
Nurses 47
   role of 100, 137
Nursing activity
   pathway 110f
   system for 109
Nursing administration 28
Nursing discharge and medical report writing 110
Nursing duty schedule 107f
Nursing informatics 26, 111
   application of 27
   limitations of 28
   need of 27
   objectives of 27
   system, purposes of 104
   theories of 28
Nursing information 103
   systems 49, 103, 111
      benefits of 112f
      components 104
   technology 112
Nursing practice 1, 27
   doctor of 140
Nursing procedures 105
Nursing records 105
Nursing staff administration 107

O

Online analytical processing 122
Online resources 4
Online searching 8
Operations domain 36
Order-entry result reporting application 53
Organizational culture 86

P

Package, total cost of 42
Patient administration 53
   management system, role of 53
Patient bed chart 57
Patient bedwise
   notification 57
   services 57
Patient care
   delivery system 1
   information system 50
      bridging of 53f
Patient consultation 58
Patient education 28
Patient generated health data 117
Patient investigation billing record 59
Patient portals 63
Patient record
   management system 64, 64f
   system 106, 106f, 107f
Patient registries 43
Patient safety 73
   and clinical risk 73
   informatics 73, 74
   outcomes, monitoring of 75
Performance analysis without hassles, process of 34
Personal data 117
Pharmacy information systems 50
Physicians 46
   information systems 49
Picture archiving and communication system 47, 115
Pivot table 22
Planning and system design 101
Poor communication 66
Population health management 124
Portal technology 68
PowerPoint, basic tasks in 23
Powers accurate medical decisions 88
Practical applications 67, 68
Practice management software 43
Predictive analytics 114
Prepare data 11
Prescriptive analytics 114
Primary care health services 35
Privacy 130, 131
Professional training 98
Protected health information 62
Provide patient-centered care 135
Public health 76, 98
   informatics 26, 95, 99
   role of 101
   programmes 101

Q

Quality
    healthcare 134
    improvement 134, 136
    transactions 69

R

Radiology information system 48, 115
Real-time
    data 29
    updates 11
Regular technology updates 75
Remote patient observation 43
Research 28
    and information, fast access to 3
Ribbon 15, 22
Risk 73
    assessment 81
    avoidance 82
    identification, sources of 78
    management 73
        process 73, 77, 78, 79f, 80f, 81
    matrix model 81f
    mitigation 73
    reduction 81
    sharing 82
Robotics 30
    process automation 69

S

Safeguarding clinical trials 123
Safety risk identification 75
Saving new document 19
Secondary care health services 35
Security 132
    principle of 130
Shareable knowledge 28
Shortcut menus 22
Social sciences, statistical package for 9
Software 2
Staff reticence 65
Stakeholder involvement 75
Standard toolbar 21
Stata 10
Statistic 2
Statistical analysis 11

Statistical packages 2, 8
    functions of 9
    types of 9
Statistical software suite 10
Storage 2
Strategic strategy 66
Study schedules 4
System manager 41
Systems theory 28

T

Tabs 22
Technical resource limitations 65
Technological aptitudes 97
Technological skill requirements 111
Technology 86
    optimization 75
Tele-health 95
Tele-medicine 6, 95
Tele-monitoring 95
Tissue 117
Training domain database 39f
Transaction data 117
Transparency, principle of 130

U

Universal health coverage 98
Use quality improvement techniques 136
Utilize informatics 136

V

Virtual private network 36
Virtual reality 30
Visualization tools 4

W

Web network 36
Web-based system 42
Webinars 91
Wizard 22
Word
    application 15
    programme 12
Workflow optimization 123
Workgroup collaboration 139

EU GSPR Authorised Reprsentative
Logos Europe, 9 rue Nicolas Poussin
1700, La Rochelle, France
Phone: +33 (0) 6 67 93 73 78
E-mail: contact@logoseurope.eu

www.ingramcontent.com/pod-product-compliance
Ingram Content Group UK Ltd.
Pitfield, Milton Keynes, MK11 3LW, UK
UKHW050428150426
5217IPUK00019B/1299